The Mediterranean Diet for Beginners 2022

A Step-by-Step Complete Beginner's Guide.100+ Easy and Quick Healthy and Delicious Recipes with a 7-Day Weight Loss Meal Plan On Mediterranean

By Asher Aiden

Table of Contents

Introduction

The Mediterranean diet incorporates items from every major food group, and there is no shortage of options that are fresh, healthy, natural, and unprocessed. Even if certain components are given more weight than others, natural ones are not ignored.

Members of the Mediterranean diet community may enjoy their favorite dishes while learning to recognize the health benefits of the purest, most natural ingredients.

Mediterranean diets may be traced back to the early inhabitants of the Mediterranean coasts of Greece, Italy, Spain, Morocco, and France.

The climates in question are classified as mild, therefore fresh seasonal produce and seafood are relied upon for sustenance most of the year.Visualizing your meals as if it were always summer is the simplest strategy to acquire a handle on the ideas underlying the Mediterranean diet.It may also trigger a sense of nostalgia for the beach fare or other summertime treats that you enjoyed most.To be honest, following a Mediterranean food plan is never boring.The Mediterranean diet is a great way to meet new people, and it may also help you rediscover the pleasure of eating by letting you know that the food you are eating is the healthiest option.Keeping up with the trends is straightforward and exciting when your diet makes you feel like you're constantly on vacation. If you've been living under a rock for the last several years, you're probably familiar with the Mediterranean diet. The popularity of this diet has been steadily growing over the last several years, and for good reason. When considering nutritional density and convenience, many people go to the Mediterranean diet (often called the heart-healthy diet).

Unchained Mediterranean diet

When one examines it more closely, the Mediterranean diet is not what one would expect from a diet designed to help with weight loss. The Mediterranean diet is more of a cultural norm and a culinary heritage for people who live in that area. This eating plan centers on whole, unrefined grains; seasonal produce; wild or farmed seafood; almonds; olive oil; and a few glasses of red wine once in a while. The food of the Mediterranean region is typical of a culture that puts a lot of value on fresh, locally grown ingredients that are cooked in a simple but tasty way and shared with loved ones over a casual meal.

Even while most of us understand the importance of eating a good, balanced diet for our health and well-being, only a minority of us really put this knowledge into practice.

Since most of our waking hours are spent at work, most of us prefer to go for quick and simple options when it comes to the food that we eat.

As a result of their low prices and high convenience, fast food, frozen meals from the grocery store, and processed foods are often our go-to options. People no longer eat according to the seasons as much as they used to because there are grocery stores open all year round. Also, making a delicious dinner from scratch takes a lot of time, and our schedules are already full, so it seems like an unnecessary hassle. Because of this, instead of eating food that grows on plants, people eat food that is made inside plants. Most of us cannot even accurately pronounce the names of the artificial additives that are a staple in our meals, nor can we identify them by sight.One of the most enticing aspects of the Mediterranean diet is that it is not difficult in any way.You don't have to be a master chef to make some of the best dishes thanks to the recipes in this area.Reduce your intake of red meat and increase your intake of fish, especially fatty fish that are high in omega-3 fatty acids; replace other oils with extra virgin olive oil when cooking; and snack often on fresh produce, whole grains, nuts, and nut butters. Cutting down on red meat and increasing your fish intake may lower your risk of cardiovascular disease.Olive oil, salmon, avocados, almonds, and seeds are all examples of healthy fats that are featured prominently in the Mediterranean diet. That's in contrast to the countless diet trends that come and go.In addition, a few glasses of red wine here and there may help lower the risk of cardiovascular disease.

Mediterranean Eating's Origins

Those who are in tune with nature and their sense of taste may find nourishment in the Mediterranean heritage of cuisine that is rich in flavor, color, and pleasant memories.

Although the Mediterranean diet has been widely covered in the media, only a minority of people really adhere to its strict guidelines.

Some people think that pizza is the most important part of the Mediterranean diet, while others think that pasta with meat sauce is the most important thing.

In this book, we'll look at where the Mediterranean diet came from so we can understand its parts better. This diet is great for your heart because it comes from the Mediterranean basin. The Mediterranean basin is also known as "The Cradle of Society" because all of the history of the ancient world happened within its borders.However, the history of where the Mediterranean diet really originated is unknown.It's possible that we'll revert to the diets of the Middle Ages or even farther back to the Romans, whose agrarian civilization was represented by red wine, bread, and oil. The cultural norms of the Roman Empire were based on those of the Greeks.Humans in the Mediterranean region often subsisted not just on the bounty of the sea but also on the fruits, vegetables, and other foods they grew on their farms.This region did not produce a lot of beef or dairy because of the poor grazing conditions brought on by the weather.Back then, seafood, goats, and lambs were the most common sources of meat protein.

Mediterranean diet science

The Mediterranean diet is often known as the "hearthealthy diet" for good reason. Fresh fruits and vegetables, whole grains, and beans take center stage on this time-honored eating plan, while fatty fish and low-fat dairy products are consumed in moderation, and meat, saturated fat, and added sugar are strictly limited.

The fats in this diet come mostly from olive oil, avocado, salmon, nuts, and seeds.

Consumption of red wine, an alcoholic beverage, is kept to a minimum.

Studies in the 1960s found that men who followed a normal Mediterranean diet had fewer instances of heart attacks, and therefore the phrase "heart-healthy diet" was established to describe such a diet. Due to this, the diet plan was developed.

Further studies have indicated that a diet comparable to the Mediterranean diet is associated with a lower incidence of stroke, cardiovascular disease, type 2 diabetes, and premature death due to health issues.

Following the rules of the Mediterranean diet has also been shown to help people think better.

A lot of research has shown that the link between the Mediterranean diet and dementia is a good one.

The high antioxidant content of the Mediterranean diet is due in large part to the eating of fresh fruit and vegetables and the occasional use of red wine.

These antioxidants have shown promise in protecting against age-related cognitive decline. These antioxidants may also increase levels of a protein that helps shield brain cells from damage.

Inflammation is a major factor in the development of Alzheimer's disease, and it is well recognized that a diet high in olive oil, fish, and fruits and vegetables may help reduce inflammation in the body.

Many of us have found that following a Mediterranean diet is the most cost-effective way to guarantee that we will always be in peak physical condition.

Mediterranean Diet Health and Longevity

The Mediterranean diet may be regarded one of the keys to finding the fountain of youth due to its focus on whole, unprocessed, natural, healthy, and freshly prepared foods. The positive effects of this diet on your appearance and energy levels will become immediately apparent as soon as you commit to it and start following it. Following the Mediterranean diet now may pay off in better health in the future.

Why Eat Mediterranean?
Fewer processed meals and no added sweeteners

The Mediterranean diet is based on olive oil, peas, beans, fruits, nuts, seeds, vegetables, and unprocessed whole grain products. It encourages eating food as close to its natural state as possible.

Wild-caught fish, especially sardines, salmon, and anchovies, are a popular alternative to plant-based diets.

Yogurts and cheeses produced by goats, cows, or sheep are great sources of calcium, healthy fats, and good cholesterol if consumed in moderation.
Even though most individuals in the Mediterranean region are not vegans, this diet recommends eating very little meat.
Choose to eat and drink things that are beneficial for your health and will help you slim down.

Safe and long-term weight loss

If you want to trim down without becoming hungry and keep the weight off permanently without making any substantial adjustments to your routine, this is the diet for you.

Many individuals have lost weight and improved their health by following this diet, which places less emphasis on processed meals and more on plant-based foods to get rid of bad fats. It has also been shown to aid with weight loss.

The Mediterranean diet can also be changed to fit your tastes for protein, carbs, or a mix of both.

Fruit, vegetables, healthy fats, and high-quality protein sources are the most important parts of the Mediterranean diet.

The advantages to your heart health are enhanced.
The Mediterranean diet relies heavily on olive oil. There is evidence that a compound found in olive oil called alpha-linoleic acid may reduce the chance of death from cardiovascular problems by as much as 45 percent.

A lower risk of mortality from cardiovascular disease is associated with eating a Mediterranean diet high in foods rich in omega-3 and monounsaturated fats. This is because the diet reduces both hypertension and harmful cholesterol.

It tirelessly fends off cancer.
The Mediterranean diet, which includes the use of olive oil, fruit, vegetables, and wine, is beneficial because it delivers a sufficient amount of omega-3 and omega-6 essential fats, as well as fiber, vitamins,

antioxidants, minerals, and polyphenols. The ideal ratio of omega-3 to omega-6 fats is also encouraged in the Mediterranean diet.A diet full of antioxidants helps fight cancer from every angle. It protects DNA, reduces inflammation, stops cell mutation, and delays the growth of tumors.

Research also suggests that olive oil might help lower your colon and bowel cancer risk.

Reduces the risk of developing diabetes and improves current symptoms.

When it comes to lowering systemic inflammation, no diet beats the Mediterranean diet for its emphasis on whole, natural ingredients.

This anti-inflammatory property aids the fight against chronic diseases like type 2 diabetes, which are linked to inflammation.
Due to its effect on insulin levels, the Mediterranean diet helps people avoid developing diabetes. The hormone insulin controls how much sugar is in the blood, and having too much of it leads you to gain weight and store sugar and other carbohydrates as fat.

Once your blood sugar levels are under control thanks to a healthy diet, your body will be better able to burn fat.

This not only aids in keeping blood sugar levels steady, but it also has the potential to help with weight loss.

This heart-healthy eating plan is an all-natural way to keep your mind sharp, and it has been linked to a reduced risk of developing dementia, Parkinson's disease, and Alzheimer's disease, as well as fewer symptoms associated with these diseases when followed strictly.

If your brain isn't getting the fuel it needs, it can't make enough of the hormone dopamine, which is essential for regulating your mood, coordinating your muscles, and handling your thoughts.

The healthy food eaten on a Mediterranean diet not only helps to avoid the cognitive decline that comes with becoming older, but it also protects against the harmful effects of toxic material exposure.

Longevity

If you eat a diet that is fresh, nourishing, natural, organic, and healthful, your body's systems will be working at peak efficiency, and you'll have more stamina for your daily activities.

Your hair and skin will both benefit from this.

You'll feel as fresh and rejuvenated as if you were just born again.

Excellent for relieving stress and unwinding.

The Mediterranean way of life is comprised of more than just eating healthy food; it also stresses the value of spending time in nature and with those who are most important to you, such as your family and friends.

The best way to spend time with loved ones is to have a delicious and healthy home-cooked meal outside, surrounded by nature, while cracking jokes and doing things that everyone enjoys.

Perhaps even start dancing.

Having a glass of red wine with loved ones after dinner is the perfect ending to the day.

If you adopt the Mediterranean diet and way of life, you will feel more at peace with yourself, have better overall health, and be able to maintain a healthy weight with less effort.This experience will teach you how to appreciate nature and everything it has to offer on a much deeper level.

Mediterranean diet

It is now beyond any shadow of a doubt that the Mediterranean diet is not a fad diet whose catchy name would help you lose ten pounds in one week. This plan, which can be summed up as a "common sense approach to eating and living," will improve your health, quality of life, and general well-being. One of the many reasons this diet is so user-friendly and easy is that it does not ban the use of any of the primary food groups.

This diet plan is also quite affordable.

Now, let's take a look at a simple method for adopting this diet and seeing its heart-healthy benefits for ourselves.

Following the Mediterranean Diet

When it comes to the Mediterranean diet, there is no one "correct" approach. That there are many different countries in the Mediterranean region, each with its own unique food culture, should be proof enough that there is no "one size fits all" approach to taking on this diet. Keep your plate mostly plant-based, with fruits and vegetables making up the bulk of your meal. Try eating fish at least twice a week, and keep red meat to once a week at most. Legumes and whole grains are two more super-healthy food groups that deserve a spot on your menu. You may create a nutritious and tasty snack out of seeds and nuts, and you should always use olive oil while cooking.

Experts suggest that people on the Mediterranean diet consume at least eight glasses of water every day.

One glass of red wine with dinner is good for your heart.

A Mediterranean diet shopping list

- You should prioritize fewer processed foods, giving more weight to fresh, organic options when available. Do most of your grocery shopping at the store's outer edges, where you are more likely to find whole meals.
Here's a short shopping list to keep in mind the next time you have to stock up on groceries: Grapes, apples, berries, citrus fruits, avocados, bananas, papayas, pineapples, etc. are all examples of fruits.
- Vegetables include, but are not limited to, broccoli, mushrooms, celery, carrots, kale, onions, leeks, eggplant, and many more.
- Mixed frozen veggies are a healthy alternative. Beans, lentils, peas, and other legumes.
- Whole-grain products, such as pasta and bread, are recommended. Nuts of many kinds, including but not limited to the aforementioned.
- variety of seeds: pumpkin, hemp, sesame, sunflower, etc.
- There are many different kinds of fish in the ocean, like salmon, tuna, herring, sardines, sea bass, and many others.
- Other shellfish and shrimp
- Chickens raised without confinement
- Small and large sweet potatoes
- Cheese
- authentic Greek yogurt

- Olives
- Grass-fed eggs
- Meat from pastured pigs, goats, and cows.
- Virgin olive oil that hasn't been processed
- To follow the principles of the Mediterranean diet, you need to get rid of everything unhealthy in your home kitchen. Candy, crackers, sodas, and other beverages containing artificial sweeteners and refined grain products are all examples of such processed foods.

If you just stock your kitchen with nutritious options, that's what you'll eat.

What isn't on the table won't be eaten.

Mediterranean Diet Dining Suggestions

A Mediterranean diet may be followed with little effort in most restaurants.
Consume seafood or fish as your primary meal.
Soak your bread in extra virgin olive oil and fry your dish in it.

Butter is bad for you, so swap it out for extra virgin olive oil on your whole wheat toast.

Relax with a glass of red wine and some sweet fruit like berries or grapes.

So, we've covered every principle of the Mediterranean diet, and now we can get to the good stuff: the food!

Put on your apron and help me prepare dinner!

7- Days Meal Plan

Here is a sample menu for a week on the Mediterranean diet.

Monday

Breakfast: The first meal of the day was strawberry Greek yogurt topped with chia seeds and Greek yogurt.

Lunch: For lunch, I had a sandwich that I had made with whole grain bread, hummus, and various vegetables.

Dinner: A fruit salad and a tuna salad that included leaves and olive oil were served for dinner. The tuna salad also had some fruit.

Tuesday

Breakfast: Make oats with blueberries for breakfast.

Lunch: a Caprese salad made with zucchini noodles, olive oil, balsamic vinegar, mozzarella, and cherry tomatoes.

Dinner: To round up the meal, a salad with feta cheese, grilled chicken, tomatoes, olives, and cucumbers was served.

Wednesday

Breakfast: I'm going to enjoy a veggie omelet with a side of toast for breakfast.

Lunch: Lunch consists of a sandwich prepared with whole-grain bread, cheese, and other raw vegetables.

Dinner: For supper, I made lasagna with a Mediterranean twist.

Thursday

Breakfast: Breakfast of yogurt topped with sliced fruit and almonds

Lunch: The chickpea and quinoa salad is what we'll be eating for lunch.

Dinner: Cooked salmon will be served on a bed of brown rice and grilled vegetables.

Friday

Breakfast: Breakfast consists of eggs, vegetables sautéed in butter, and whole wheat toast.

Lunch: For lunch, we will be having pesto-filled zucchini boats stuffed with turkey sausage, tomatoes, bell peppers, and cheese.

Dinner: Dinner of grilled lamb skewers, salad, and baked potatoes

Saturday

Breakfast: The morning meal was a bowl of porridge with apple slices, raisins, and almonds sprinkled on top.

Lunch: on whole wheat toast, with fresh vegetables on top.

Dinner: Our supper was a Mediterranean pizza made with whole wheat pita bread and topped with cheese, vegetables, and olives.

Sunday

Breakfast: For breakfast, I made an omelette packed with veggies and olives.

Lunch: Lunch was a plate of falafel accompanied by hummus, rice, feta cheese, onions, tomatoes, and hummus.

Dinner: For dinner, we had grilled chicken with a selection of vegetables, sweet potato fries, and fruit salad.

My Recipes

Recipe : Cauliflower Rabe With Hot Garlic

Prep Time : 0 Hour 2 Minutes

Total Time : 0 Hour 10 Minutes

Yields: 4 Servings

Material :

- 2 tablespoons of high-quality olive oil 1 1/2 pounds of broccoli rabe.
- three cloves garlic
- About a quarter of a teaspoon of crushed red pepper flakes

Step :

- If you want your broccoli rabe to be crisp-tender but still have a bite to it, cut the stem ends and simmer it in boiling, salted water for two to three minutes. We recommend a good drainage system. Cook the garlic for two to three minutes in a large pan over medium heat with a generous amount of extra-virgin olive oil. A soft browning of the garlic is desired. Toss in some crushed spicy red pepper flakes and give the dish another 30 seconds in the cooking pot. Cook the broccoli rabe for another two minutes after adding it, stirring it around the pan often.

Recipe : Chickpea-tomato stew with ginger

Prep Time : 0 Hour 15 Minutes

Total Time : 0 Hour 40 Minutes

Yields: 4 Servings

Material :

- 2 tablespoons of oil from a vegetable source.
  The equivalent of one large onion
  In this case, we'll need 2 garlic cloves.
- 1.25 oz. of basmati rice
- Approximately 1 cup of low-fat plain yogurt.
- Approximately one-fourth cup of fresh cilantro
  leaves, securely packed
- Cumin powder, 2 milligrams
- A pinch of ground coriander, or 1 teaspoon
- Half a teaspoon of dried oregano.
- 1 can chopped tomatoes
- Fresh lemon juice, 2 tbsp.
- sliced fresh ginger, one tablespoon's worth of
  grated
- 3 cups ready-to-eat garbanzo beans
- half a cup of water
- Sugar, about 1 1/2 teaspoons
- salt
- Pappadums

Step :

- Heat the oil in a 5-to 6-quart saucepot over medium heat until it is hot. Add the onions and garlic and combine. Stir the veggies occasionally for ten minutes, until they are golden brown and tender.
- Rice should be prepared in accordance with package instructions. Combine the yogurt and cilantro in a small bowl and mix to blend. Cover and refrigerate the cilantro yogurt until ready to use.
  The onion should already be in the saucepot when you add the cumin, coriander, and ground red pepper. Stir for 1 minute, or until the scent is released. The recipe needs tomatoes, lemon juice, and ginger. Toss in some garbanzo beans and some water and let everything come to a boil together. Simmer for 15–20 minutes, mashing some of the beans occasionally, until the sauce reaches the desired thickness. Combine the sugar and salt, about a quarter of a teaspoon. Around 7 cups may be obtained from this recipe.
- Distribute some rice to each serving dish. Arrange the bean and yogurt mixture in a layer above the garnish. Pappadums are optional with this meal.

Recipe : tomato couscous

Prep Time : 0 Hour 10 Minutes

Total Time : 0 Hour 15 Minutes

Yields: 4   Servings

Material :

- 4 large plum tomatoes. single cup of grape or cherry tomatoes,
  1 packet pearled couscous scented with basil and herbs
- 14 cup of water1 tablespoon extra virgin olive oil
- Fresh lemon juice, 2 tbsp.
- Cheese Parmesan, 2 oz.
- 1.5 ounces of prosciutto.
- Toasted pine nuts, about a quarter cup

Step :

- Prepare the couscous as directed on the box. Using a whisk, mix the lemon juice, olive oil, and a half teaspoon each of kosher salt and freshly ground pepper to make the vinaigrette.
- Slice beefsteak tomatoes in half lengthwise, scoop out the pulp and seeds, then sprinkle the cut surfaces with coarse salt.
- After the couscous has cooked, transfer it to a large bowl and toss it with the vinaigrette. Mix in the pine nuts, the prosciutto, the Parmesan,

and the cherry tomatoes, and toss again. Use a spoon to fill the tomatoes with the mixture. Serve with flatbread crackers and garnished with fresh basil leaves.

Recipe : Eggplant Cilantro Dip

Prep Time : 0 Hour 10 Minutes

Total Time : 0 Hour 55 Minutes

Yields: 1 Servings

Material :

- This is the equivalent of 2 whole eggplants.
  Four garlic cloves,
  The equivalent of 3 tablespoons of tahini
- A squeeze of lemon, about 3 tablespoons' worth
- salt
- Loosely packed fresh cilantro or mint leaves,
  1/4 cup
- toasty, grilled pita slices.
- Snacks of raw vegetables, such as carrot and
  cucumber sticks and sliced red or yellow
  peppers,

Step :

- Bake at 450 degrees Fahrenheit until the
  temperature is raised. Nonstick foil should be
  used to line a jelly-roll pan measuring 15 1/2 by
  10 1/2 inches (or use regular foil and spray
  with nonstick cooking spray). Place the eggplant
  halves in the foil-lined pan, skin side up. It's best
  to cook the garlic alongside the eggplants by
  wrapping the cloves in foil and then placing
  them in the pan. Cook the vegetables in the oven
  for 45–50 minutes, or until the eggplants are

soft and the skin has shrunk and browned. Rub the garlic with a peeler. When working with garlic or eggplant, wait until they have cooled enough to handle comfortably.

- Once the eggplants have cooled, you may remove the flesh and place it in a food processor equipped with a knife blade. Squeeze the pulp from the garlic cloves and add them to the food processor along with the tahini, lemon juice, and 3/4 of a teaspoon of salt. Put the ingredients in the machine and pulse it a few times to coarsely chop them. Put the dip in a serving bowl and stir in the cilantro. Refrigerate for at least two hours after covering and chilling. Along with the pita bread, serve with the dip.

Recipe : Hazelnut-glazed carrots

Prep Time : 0 Hour 25 Minutes

Total Time : 0 Hour 25 Minutes

Yields: 4 Servings

Material :

- 2 tbsp. butter.
  2 milligrams shredded orange rind
- 1/4 c. juice of an orange
- a splash of dry white wine, about 2 tablespoons
- 2 tbsp. a sweetener made from maple trees
- half a cup coarsely chopped roasted hazelnuts

Step :

- In a large frying pan, melt the butter and sauté the carrots, stirring them every so often, until they are almost done.
  Then, add the rind, juice, wine, and syrup, and bring to a boil. Cover the carrots and keep cooking them over low heat for about 20 minutes, or until all the liquid has evaporated and the carrots are soft and caramelized.
  Serve carrots with a nut topping.

Recipe : Vinaigrette

Prep Time : 0 Hour 10 Minutes

Total Time : 0 Hour 10 Minutes

Yields: 4 Servings

Material :

- 1/2 cup of high-quality olive oil.
  One-fourth of a cup of red wine vinegar.
  1 garlic clove, minced and peeled
- Ketchup, 1 tablespoon
- 12 tsp of coarsely grated lemon peel.
- 2 ml of freshly squeezed lemon juice.
- Granulated sugar, 2 teaspoons
- Kosher salt, one teaspoon.
- Brand-new, freshly ground black pepper, 1 teaspoon.
- As an example, consider 1 tsp of Worcestershire sauce.

Step :

- Combine all of the ingredients in a medium-sized bowl and stir until uniformly blended.

Recipe : Peppers, Grilled

Prep Time : 0 Hour 15Minutes

Total Time : 0 Hour 22 Minutes

Yields: 6 Servings

Material :

- Four peppers of varying colors: red, orange, yellow
  Extra virgin olive oil, two teaspoons, a pinch of salt, half a tsp.
- Peppercorns, around 1/4 milligram in size, are made from black pepper.
- Parsley, about a quarter cup's worth

Step :

- Prepare an outside grill for direct grilling over a medium fire.
  Before slicing each pepper in half lengthwise, remove the stem and any seeds. In a medium bowl, mix the peppers, oil, half a teaspoon of salt, and a quarter of a teaspoon of roughly powdered black pepper.
- Arrange the peppers, skin-side up, on the grill rack. Grill the peppers for about four to five minutes with the lid closed, or until they become malleable. Turn the peppers over, cover, and let them simmer for another three to four minutes, or until they have a light char.

Return the cooked peppers to the bowl. Serve with a generous helping of minced parsley.

Recipe : Chimichurri-Riced Shrimp

Prep Time : 0 Hour 15 Minutes

Total Time : 0 Hour 25 Minutes

Yields: 4   Servings

Material :

- a medium-sized orange and one cup of long-grain rice
  1 cup cilantro leaves, freshly chopped
- The equivalent of 4 scallions
- In this case, we'll need 2 garlic cloves.
- 2 teaspoons extra virgin olive oil
- a pinch of red pepper flakes
- fine sea salt.
- Pepper
- 1 pound of shrimp
- One-half a milligram of cumin powder
- One avocado

Step :

- Cook the rice according to the package's directions. While that is happening, zest two oranges and grate them finely. Segment the orange while standing over a large bowl to avoid dropping any of the segments into the basin. Remove the skin and the white pith with a sharp knife. Firstly, you should rough-chop the segments before putting them in the bowl. Squeeze the membrane's contents into a dish, then add the other ingredients (the cilantro, scallions, garlic, 1 tbsp oil, 1/4 tsp salt, and the red pepper flakes).

- A single tablespoon of oil should be heated in a big pan over medium heat. Cumin, a quarter teaspoon each of salt and pepper, and the reserved zest from earlier should be used to season the shrimp. Stir the mixture every minute or two for three to four minutes, or until it is completely opaque all over.

Once the avocado and rice have been mixed with the chimichurri sauce, the shrimp may be added.

Recipe : The Chicken Caprese

Prep Time : 0 Hour 10 Minutes

Total Time : 0 Hour 30 Minutes

Yields: 4   Servings

Material :

- Chicken breasts without the skin and bones that weigh one pound with Kosher salt
- cracked black pepper that has just been ground.
- 1/4 cup balsamic vinegar
- 2 minced or chopped garlic cloves.
- 1 oz. halved grape tomatoes
- 1 bunch of fresh basil, torn into 2 teaspoons.
- Four pieces of fresh mozzarella,

Step :

- To heat the oil, place a large skillet over medium heat. Grill the chicken for 6 minutes on each side, or until browned and cooked through, after seasoning with salt and pepper. Arrangement on a serving plate and put away.
- Once the garlic has been in the pan for a minute, drizzle in the balsamic vinegar and toss to incorporate. Once the tomatoes are added, salt to taste. Let it cook for 5–7 minutes, or until tender. Add some basil and mix it up. Reheat the chicken and then top it with the

tomatoes in the pan. Cover the dish with the lid
and sprinkle the mozzarella on top to melt.
- Tomatoes should be spooned over the chicken
after plating.

Recipe : Chickpea salad

Prep Time : 0 Hour 20 Minutes

Total Time : 0 Hour 25 Minutes

Yields: 6 Servings

Material :

- Two 15-ounce cans of chickpeas with the liquid drained and rinsed. The equivalent of one medium cucumber, chopped; one small red pepper, chopped
- half a red onion, thinly sliced
- olives, kalamata, diced, half a cup
- 0.5 tbsp crumbled feta cheese
- Kojic salt
- pepper, black, that has just been ground.
- Vinaigrete with lemon and parsley
- 1/2 cup of pure olive oil.
- White wine vinegar, measuring 1/4 cup
- 1 tablespoon of fresh lemon juice.
- Fresh parsley, chopped to equal 1 tablespoon
- The equivalent of one-fourth of a teaspoon of crushed red pepper.
- Kosher salt is a Jewish tradition.
- pepper, black, that has just been ground.

Step :

- To make the salad, mix together a big bowl's worth of chickpeas, cucumber, bell pepper, red

onion, olives, and feta. Season with salt and
pepper just before serving.

- Olive oil, vinegar, lemon juice, fresh parsley, and
crushed red pepper flakes are the main
ingredients of a classic vinaigrette. Get a good
shake out of the bottle. Season with salt and
pepper after sealing the container and shaking
the contents until they are well combined.
It's best to dress the salad with vinaigrette just
before serving.

Recipe : Salmon Greek

Prep Time : 0 Hour 20 Minutes

Total Time : 0 Hour 50 Minutes

Yields: 4   Servings

Material :

- One-fourth cup of high-quality olive oil
  The juice of two lemons
  1 garlic clove, minced
- Dried Oregano, 1 Teaspoon
- 1/2 teaspoon red pepper flakes
- pepper, black, that has just been ground.
- One cup of diced feta.
- Tomatoes, one cup, halved or quartered; or cherry tomatoes, one cup
- Kalamata olives, sliced (about a quarter of a cup)
- Iranian cucumbers, diced; 1/4 cup
- Red onion, chopped (14)
- Fresh dill, chopped (about 2 teaspoons)
- WITH SALMON
- 1 lemon, cut very thinly,
- 1 small red onion, thinly sliced
- A total of 12 ounces of salmon was cut into 4 fillets and wiped dry using paper towels.
- Kosher salt is a Jewish tradition.
- pepper, black, that has just been ground.

Step :

- Set the oven temperature to 375 degrees. Whisk together the olive oil, lemon juice, garlic, oregano, and crushed red pepper flakes in a large bowl; add the feta and let marinate for at least an hour. After coating, pepper is added, and the feta is stirred in. Put it in the fridge for approximately ten minutes while you get the rest of the ingredients ready.
Prepare a large baking dish by layering the bottom with the sliced lemon and red onion before adding the fish. Flake the salmon and lay it skin-side down in a baking dish. Bake for 18–20 minutes, or until the fish is opaque and flaky, after sprinkling with salt and pepper.
- While that's going on, throw the feta cheese in a dish with the tomatoes, olives, cucumbers, red onion, and dill for the topping. Combining ingredients requires gentle folding.
- Place the salmon on a platter, top with the lemon and onion pieces, and then sprinkle with the feta mixture.

Recipe : Garlic-tomato-mussels

Prep Time : 0 Hour 25 Minutes

Total Time : 0 Hour 25 Minutes

Yields: 4 Servings

Material :

- 1 pound of butter
  1 medium onion, chopped3 minced garlic cloves.
- a single 15-ounce chopped tomato can
- half a teaspoon of dry white wine
- Fresh parsley, chopped (about 2 teaspoons) and extra for garnish
- fine sea salt.
- pepper, black, that has just been ground.
- Mussels, 2 pounds, beards removed
- Served with grilled bread.

Step :

- Butter may be melted in a pot set over a stove burner set to medium heat. To soften and release its flavor, sauté the onion for about five minutes after adding it. Then, when the onion is soft, add the garlic and let it simmer for another minute, or until the garlic smell comes out.
  Be careful to combine the tomato chunks, wine, and parsley after adding them. Put in some pepper and salt to taste.

- You need to keep boiling the liquid for several minutes after you add the mussels, or until the shells have opened. If a shell isn't already open, toss it.
- Toast some bread and sprinkle with some more chopped parsley before serving.

Recipe : Broccolini that has been roasted

Prep Time : 0 Hour 5 Minutes

Total Time : 0 Hour 40 Minutes

Yields: 4 Servings

Material :

- 2 tablespoons extra-virgin olive oil
  Kosher salt is a Jewish tradition.
- pepper, black, that has just been ground.
- Ingredients include crushed red pepper flakes.

Step :

- Set the temperature in the oven to 425 degrees. Spread the broccoli florets in a single layer on a large baking sheet and drizzle with oil. After adding salt, pepper, and crushed red pepper flakes, toss the mixture to make sure the ingredients are evenly distributed. Wait to eat until the meat is soft enough to pierce with a fork and the ends look charred, which should take about 30 minutes in the oven.

Recipe : Salad Greek

Prep Time : 0 Hour 15 Minutes

Total Time : 0 Hour 15 Minutes

Yields: 4 Servings

Material :

- Grape or cherry tomatoes, one ounce each, halved Ingredients: 1 cucumber, cut as thinly as possible into half moons.
  1 cup Kalamata olives, halved
- Very thinly sliced half of a red onion
- A little less than three-quarters of an ounce of crumbled feta.
- used as a condiment.
- Red wine vinegar, 2 teaspoons.
- One-half of a lemon's juice
- Dried Oregano, 1 Teaspoon
- Kosher salt is a Jewish tradition.
- pepper, black, that has just been ground.
- One-fourth cup of high-quality olive oil.

Step :

- In a large bowl, toss together the chopped tomatoes, cucumbers, olives, and red onion for the salad. Use a delicate touch while mixing the feta.
- Follow these steps to make the dressing in a small bowl: After mixing together the vinegar,

lemon juice, and oregano, season with salt and pepper. Slowly drizzle in the olive oil while continuously whisking.
Dress the salad and serve.

Recipe : Swordfish steak

Prep Time : 0 Hour 10 Minutes

Total Time : 0 Hour 20 Minutes

Yields: 4 Servings

Material :

- a tablespoon of extra-virgin olive oil, kosher salt
- freshly ground black pepper.
- Cherry tomatoes of varying hues, 2 ounces each, halved
- a quarter of a red onion, coarsely chopped
- About 3 tablespoons of basil, sliced paper-thin.
- Half a lemon's worth of juice

Step :

- Crank up the temperature to 400 degrees.
  In a large, heavy-bottomed cast-iron skillet, heat the oil for two teaspoons over high heat. Season the tops of the fish fillets with salt and pepper before placing them in the pan. Three to five minutes should be enough time for the fish to brown on one side. Turn the steak over and season the other side with salt and pepper. Put the pan in the oven and remove it from the heat.
  The swordfish should be flaky and cooked through after being roasted for about 10 minutes.

- Tomatoes, onion, and basil should be combined in a big dish for the fresh tomato salad. Season with salt and pepper and squeeze in the juice of half a lemon.
- Before serving, top the salmon with the salad.

Recipe : Chicken-Stuffed Zucchini

Prep Time : 0 Hour 20 Minutes

Total Time : 0 Hour 45 Minutes

Yields: 6 Servings

Material :

- Three lengthwise-sliced zucchini; half an onion, diced; 2 tablespoons of extra-virgin olive oil
- Two minced or chopped garlic cloves.
- Two cups of cooked, shredded chicken.
- a pinch of dried oregano.
- Japanese-style kosher salt
- ground black pepper that has just been prepared.
- Chickpeas, one can (which is 15 ounces)
- Cut cherry tomatoes to equal a half cup.
- 1/2 cup kalamata olives
- One cup of crumbled feta cheese.
- 1/2 lemon
- Cucumber, around 3/4 cup, cut very coarsely
- For serving: fresh dill sprigs, chopped.

Step :

- Set the temperature to 350 degrees. Once the zucchini has been scored, the pulp may be easily removed and deposited in a bowl. Mix up the olive oil, salt, and pepper, then pour into a shallow baking dish. Put the veggies in the oven for 12–15 minutes, or until they are mostly soft. Remove from the oven and turn the broiler to high.

- Olive oil needs to be warmed in a big skillet over moderate heat. Incorporate the onion after around 5 minutes, and simmer until soft. While stirring frequently, continue cooking for another minute after adding the garlic. About 2 minutes later, add the carved-out zucchini and cook until it becomes a pale golden color. Toss the mixture often while cooking it for about 5 minutes after adding the shredded chicken and chickpeas, tomatoes, olives, and oregano, or until it reaches the desired temperature.

- Stuff the zucchini with the chicken mixture, then finish with a feta cheese topping. Bake for another 10 minutes, or until the zucchini is tender when pierced with a fork and the cheese has melted. Warm zucchini "boats" are served with fresh lemon juice, cucumber, and dill.

Recipe : Chicken Prepared in an Italian Skillet

Prep Time : 0 Hour 10 Minutes

Total Time : 0 Hour 40 Minutes

Yields: 4 Servings

Material :

- Ingredients: 2 tablespoons of extra-virgin olive oil, 1 pound of boneless, skinless chicken breasts, and a pinch of Kosher salt.
- ground black pepper that has just been prepared.
- a small onion (roughly half a medium)
- Thinly sliced red bell peppers (2)
- Approximately 2 medium-sized zucchini, cut in half lengthwise.
- Two minced or chopped garlic cloves.
- Oregano, dry, 1/2 teaspoon
- One cup of low-sodium chicken broth.
- 1 ounce crushed tomatoes (or 1 14-ounce can)
- A quarter cup of torn fresh basil.

Step :

- Warm the oil in a large skillet set over medium heat. The chicken should be seasoned with salt and pepper before being placed under the grill, and cooking time should be approximately 8 minutes per side. Set aside on a serving plate.

- After adding the onion and peppers to the pan, continue to cook them for another 5 minutes, or until they are soft. After adding the zucchini, continue to cook for three more minutes, or until it has a light sear, before adding the garlic and continuing to cook for one more minute, or until it is fragrant. Enhance the taste with some oregano.
  After you've added the broth and crushed tomatoes, you should keep the pot on high for another 10 minutes. Reintroduce the chicken to the pan and cover it with the sauce and the vegetables.
- Sprinkle some chopped basil on top just before serving.

Recipe : Halibut cooked on a grill

Prep Time : 0 Hour 5 Minutes

Total Time : 0 Hour 20 Minutes

Yields: 5 Servings

Material :

- Steaks of halibut, four servings (4-6 ounces each)
  Kosher salt and 2 tablespoons of extra-virgin olive oil
- ground black pepper that has just been prepared.
- The Mango salsa
- Diced mango
- Garlic, finely diced1 tiny red pepper.
- Half a red onion, chopped
- 1 jalapeo, minced
- 1 tbsp of chopped cilantro.
- sufficient lime juice to make one lime.
- Japanese-style kosher salt
- ground black pepper that has just been prepared.

Step :

- After seasoning the halibut with salt and pepper and brushing both sides with oil, you can throw it on a grill set to medium-high heat. Cook the halibut on the grill for about 5 minutes each side, or until it reaches an internal temperature of 140 degrees F.

- To prepare the salsa, put all of the ingredients in a medium bowl and season with salt and pepper to taste. Attempt to eat halibut with salsa.

Recipe : Asparagus oven-roasted

Prep Time : 0 Hour 5 Minutes

Total Time : 0 Hour 30 Minutes

Yields: 4 Servings

Material :

- asparagus (about 2 pounds), stalks removed. Ingredients: 3 tablespoons of extra-virgin olive oil, 1 tablespoon of kosher salt.
- ground black pepper that has just been prepared.

Step :

- Preheat the oven to 400 degrees Fahrenheit. Place the asparagus on a large baking sheet and toss with the olive oil. Sprinkle salt and pepper over it liberally.

- The meat should be tender and have a little sear after approximately 25 minutes in the oven.

Recipe : Shrimp lemon-garlic

Prep Time : 0 Hour 5 Minutes

Total Time : 0 Hour 15 Minutes

Yields: 4 Servings

Material :

- The butter will be 2 tablespoons total, with 1 tablespoon swapped out for EVOO.
  One pound of peeled and deveined medium-sized shrimp.
- Extra-thinly sliced lemon and lemon juice from 1 lemon.
- Chopped garlic from 3 whole garlic cloves.
- a pinch of dried red pepper crushed
- Japanese-style kosher salt
- a splash of dry white wine (or water), about 2 tbsp
- Garnish with fresh parsley, if desired.

Step :

- Over medium heat, combine the 1 tablespoon of butter and the olive oil in a large pan. Incorporate the crushed red pepper flakes as a last touch after adding the shrimp, lemon slices, garlic, and salt. Cooking time for each side of the shrimp should be around three minutes, with periodic tossing to achieve uniform cooking.

- Remove the pan from the heat and, while swirling continually, add the remaining butter, lemon juice, and white wine. Add salt and garnish with chopped parsley before serving.

Recipe : Salmon broiled

Prep Time : 0 Hour 10 Minutes

Total Time : 0 Hour 20 Minutes

Yields: 4   Servings

Material :

- Four fillets of salmon, each weighing in at four ounces,
  Use 1 level tablespoon of grainy mustard.
  Two entire garlic cloves, finely chopped.
- 1 tablespoon shallots, finely chopped
- Finely chop 2 teaspoons of fresh thyme leaves; save aside any extras for presentation.
- 2 tsp. of chopped fresh rosemary,
- Half a lemon's worth of juice
- i.e., kosher salt used in cooking.
- ground black pepper that has just been prepared.
- Cut the lemon into thin pieces before serving.

Step :

- Get a parchment-lined baking sheet and the broiler hot. To make the mustard spread, combine the garlic, shallot, thyme, and rosemary in a small bowl. Add the lemon juice and season with salt and pepper. After spreading the mixture on both sides of the salmon fillets, broil them for seven to eight minutes.

- Garnish with more lemon wedges and thyme leaves before serving.

Recipe : Salmon Bowl

Prep Time : 0 Hour 20 Minutes

Total Time : 01 Hour 0 Minutes

Yields: 4 Servings

Material :

- For the salmon, use a third of a cup of low-sodium soy sauce.
  1/3 cup of high-quality olive oil.
- splash of chili garlic sauce, about a quarter cup
- sufficient lime juice to make one lime.
- Two Tablespoons of Honey
- Four minced whole garlic cloves.
- Four fillets of salmon, each weighing in at four ounces,
- In order to get ready-to-eat pickled cucumbers
- 1/2 cup rice vinegar (or rice wine vinegar)
- A total of 1 tablespoon of granulated sugar
- Salt, kosher: 1 pinch
- 12 teaspoons of roasted sesame oil
- Three Persian cucumbers, sliced paper thin
- In order to prepare the Smoking Mayonnaise
- 1/2 cup mayonnaise
- 2 tbsp. Sriracha
- 2 teaspoons of sesame oil, roasted
- With respect to the bowl
- Brown rice is rice made from brown rice.
- 1 avocado, sliced
- One medium-sized shredded carrot.

- Chopped red onion, cilantro leaves, and smashed sesame seeds are all good options.
- shredded cilantro leaves.
- Seeds of the Sesame Tree

Step :

- First, preheat the oven to 350 degrees Fahrenheit, and then line a large baking sheet with foil. In a medium bowl, whisk together the chili garlic sauce, honey, lime juice, garlic, and olive oil. Toss in the fish and gently combine the ingredients. After arranging the salmon on the prepared baking sheet, bake for 20 to 25 minutes, or until the fish flakes easily with a fork.

- Pickle some cucumbers while it's going on: In a microwave-safe jar or bowl, combine the vinegar, sugar, and salt and heat on high for about two minutes, or until the sugar and salt are dissolved. Add the cucumbers and shake the container well before adding the sesame oil. Make sure the container has a tight-fitting lid or is wrapped in plastic until it's time to use.
  Stir together some mayonnaise, Sriracha, and sesame oil to create a spicy mayo.
- Distribute the rice evenly among the four bowls, then assemble the bowls. You may garnish this dish with salmon, pickled cucumbers, avocado,

carrot, red onion, cilantro, and sesame seeds.
Drizzle some spicy mayonnaise on top.

Recipe : Arugula Caprese

Prep Time : 0 Hour 10 Minutes

Total Time : 0 Hour 30 Minutes

Yields: 6 Servings

Material :

- The equivalent of one pound of asparagus with its stems removed
Use extra-virgin olive oil to dress a salad, then finish with a sprinkle of kosher salt.
- ground black pepper that has just been prepared.
- 2 cups shredded mozzarella
- 4 medium-sized tomatoes, sliced in half.
- Half a Cup of Balsamic Vinegar
- a quarter cup of honey
- Using extremely thinly sliced fresh basil as a garnish

Step :

- Heat the oven to 425 degrees. Before baking, asparagus should be coated in olive oil, then seasoned with salt and pepper. Mozzarella should be sprinkled over the empty space on the baking sheet.

- In the other half of the baking sheet, toss cherry tomatoes with olive oil and season with salt and pepper. The asparagus should be tender and the cheese should have melted after around 20 minutes in the oven.

Meanwhile, make the balsamic glaze by combining honey and balsamic vinegar in a small saucepan. Reduce the liquid by half, about 15 minutes at a simmer while stirring occasionally (the mixture should coat the back of a spoon). Allow it to cool down a little.

- Arrange the asparagus spears with cheese on a serving dish. roasted tomatoes with a drizzle of balsamic glaze and a sprinkling of fresh basil.

Recipe : Salmon-Bruschetta

Prep Time : 0 Hour 10 Minutes

Total Time : 0 Hour 25 Minutes

Yields: 4   Servings

Material :

- A total of 4 salmon fillets, each weighing in at 6 ounces, a pinch of dried oregano Japanese-style kosher salt
- ground black pepper that has just been prepared.
- 12 cups of virgin olive oil.
- Chopped garlic from 3 whole garlic cloves.
- Two shallots, minced to a fine consistency.
- Approximately 3 cups of cherry tomatoes, halved and sliced.
- Half a lemon's worth of juice
- A quarter cup of thinly chopped basil leaves.
- Freshly grated Parmesan cheese is used in many dishes.
- Drizzleable balsamic glaze

Step :

- The salmon should be seasoned all over with oregano, salt, and pepper.
Olive oil needs to be warmed in a big skillet over moderate heat. Salmon with the skin up should be added to the pan when the oil is shimmering

but not smoking, and cooked for approximately six minutes, or until deeply browned. Flip the salmon over and continue cooking for another six minutes until it is opaque and flakes easily. Set aside on a serving plate.

- The shallots and garlic should be added to the same pan as the chicken, and the remaining tablespoon of olive oil should be stirred in. The garlic's scent will develop after it has been cooked for around a minute. After incorporating the tomatoes, add salt and pepper to taste. If you want to get the most flavor out of your tomatoes, slow cooking with frequent stirring is the way to go. Take the pan off the heat and pour some lemon juice over the top.
- On top of each serving of salmon, spoon some of the tomato sauce. After plating, sprinkle each serving with basil and Parmesan and drizzle with balsamic glaze.

Recipe : Orzo salad

Prep Time : 0 Hour 20 Minutes

Total Time : 0 Hour 35 Minutes

Yields: 5 Servings

Material :

- Two tablespoons of freshly squeezed lemon juice.
  Approximately half a teaspoon of Dijon mustard
- Extra-virgin olive oil, 1/4 cup
- Two tablespoons of fresh dill, chopped coarsely; save extra for serving.
- 14 cups of finely chopped red onion
- Japanese-style kosher salt
- ground black pepper that has just been prepared.
- Orzo, 8 oz.
- thin slices of three Persian cucumbers, formed into half-moons.
- 4 medium-sized tomatoes, sliced in half.
- A single can of chickpeas, drained and rinsed (approximately 15.5 ounces),
- olives, kalamata, 1/2 cup, halved, pitted
- One cup of feta cheese, crumbled (about 14 of a pound).

Step :

- Bring a pot of salted water to a boil and add the orzo, cooking it according to the package directions until it reaches the "al dente" stage. Set aside after rinsing.
Mix the lemon juice and mustard in a large bowl with a whisk until the dressing is creamy. Add the oil slowly while continuing to whisk until it is well absorbed. Then, add some dill and red onion and mix well before seasoning with salt and pepper.

- In a large bowl, combine the orzo, cucumbers, cherry tomatoes, chickpeas, and olives with the dressing. Toss it into the coat. If you want, you can sprinkle more dill on top after the feta has been added.

Recipe : Red Snapper

Prep Time : 0 Hour 30 Minutes

Total Time : 0 Hour 50 Minutes

Yields: 4   Servings

Material :

- 1/4 cup of chopped fresh parsley, extra-virgin olive oil, 3 teaspoons
  Finely chopped fresh oregano, one tablespoon
- A single lemon that has been sliced lengthwise, zest removed, and peeled.
- Chopped garlic from 3 whole garlic cloves.
- Two one-pound red snapper, gutted, scaled, and ready to cook.
- with freshly ground black pepper and salt to taste.

Step :

- Put the oregano, garlic, lemon zest, and olive oil in a small bowl and stir in the chopped parsley.
- It is necessary to clean the red snappers by hand and pat them dry with paper towels. Make three diagonal cuts across the top of each fish, almost to the bone, using a sharp knife. The cavities should be seasoned with salt and pepper.

- Be careful to get some of the parsley mixture inside the slits and rub it all over the inside and exterior of the fish. Position the fish so that it is in the centre of the grill pan and season it with salt and pepper.

- Select "Auto Cook" from the Panasonic Countertop Induction Oven's menu after the grill plate is in place. We recommend the fish (level 3) in the 1 lb. serving size. Cook for about 20 minutes, or until an instant-read thermometer inserted in the center registers at least 130 degrees Fahrenheit (54 degrees Celsius). Adapt the timing to your needs. Prepare the dish with slices of lemon.

Recipe : Mediterranean grilling

Prep Time : 0 Hour 15 Minutes

Total Time : 0 Hour 25 Minutes

Yields: 6 Servings

Material :

- Two Tablespoons of Olive Oil
  Balsamic vinegar, 1 teaspoon
  One Lemon juice dropperful
- 14 tsp of dried rosemary
- Oregano, in its dried form, equal to 12 teaspoons
- Cut eight large mushrooms in half or quarters.
- a large zucchini, cut into quarters
- "A large green bell pepper, split into strips
- 1 large red onion, halved and finely chopped

Step :

- Get an outside grill nice and hot before you use it.
  Olive oil, balsamic vinegar, lemon juice, rosemary, and oregano should be mixed together in a basin. Stir well to combine.

- To prepare the vegetables for grilling, brush them with the oil mixture and set them in a deep pan.

Soft meat may be achieved by cooking it for 10–15 minutes with the pan flipped over once.

Recipe : Mediterranean Chickpea Salad

Prep Time : 0 Hour 10 Minutes

Total Time : 0 Hour 10 Minutes

Yields: 4 Servings

Material :

- one-quarter cup olive oil
  For every 4 cups of red wine, use 1 cup of vinegar.
  1-tablespoon of dried oregano
- Chopped garlic equals 1 tablespoon.
- drained and rinsed, 1 15-ounce can of chickpeas
- A 6-ounce (one can's worth) of baby black olives, drained and rinsed
- Artichoke hearts, marinated, drained, 1 (6-ounce) can
- 1 jar of chopped roasted red peppers (equivalent to 6 ounces),
- 3 ounces of crumbled feta cheese.
- 1 1/2 tablespoons of non-pareil capers, cleaned and dried
- Grape leaves, or dolmas, 1 jar, drained and rinsed and ready to use (Optional)

Step :

- Dressing may be made by mixing together oil, vinegar, oregano, and garlic in a small basin.

- Mix together the chickpeas, olives, artichoke hearts, roasted red peppers, feta cheese, and capers in a big bowl. When you've finished dressing the salad, toss it. Alternatively, dolmas may be served with the meal.

Recipe : Chicken Med-Lemon

Prep Time : 0 Hour 15 Minutes

Total Time : 01 Hour 5 Minutes

Yields: 6 Servings

Material :

- 1 lemon
  oregano, dry, 2 teaspoons
  3-garlic cloves, chopped
- 2 tablespoons butter
- A pinch of salt
- A sprinkle of ground black pepper is equal to
  1/4 teaspoon.
- The equivalent of six chicken legs

Step :

- Pre-heat the oven to 425 degrees Fahrenheit
  (220 degrees Celsius).
  Half of the lemon should be grated and added to
  a 9-by-13-inch baking dish together with the
  oregano, garlic, oil, salt, and pepper. Extract
  about a quarter cup of juice from half a lemon.
  Whisk them together completely.

- The skin of any chicken pieces you use should
  be thrown away. Sprinkle the bone-side-up
  chicken pieces with salt and pepper, then coat
  them in the lemon mixture. Put the dish in the
  oven and bake it, covered, for 20 minutes.

Battered and flipped chicken.

- Continue roasting the chicken uncovered for approximately 30 minutes more after reducing the heat to 400 degrees Fahrenheit (205 degrees Celsius), basting every 10 minutes. The chicken tastes best when served with the pan juices.

Recipe : Veggie Stew

Prep Time : 0 Hour 5 Minutes

Total Time : 0 Hour 15 Minutes

Yields: 6 Servings

Material :

- Red onion, minced finely (1 cup) 2 cups of green pepper, coarsely chopped; 2 tablespoons of olive oil.
- Approximately two large garlic cloves, crushed and chopped.
- A cup of water and 1 ounce of chopped mushrooms.
- Cut one small eggplant into pieces between one and two inches in length, peel it, and set it aside.
- One 28-ounce can of crushed tomatoes.
- a half cup sliced and pitted kalamata olives
- drained and rinsed 15 ounces (1 can) of chickpeas
- Fresh, chopped rosemary, one tablespoon.
- A tablespoon of finely chopped parsley.

Step :

- Get 1 tablespoon of oil hot in a deep skillet. The onion and pepper just need around 10 minutes to soften. Toss together a tablespoon of oil, a single garlic clove, some mushrooms, and some eggplant. Don't give the mixture the occasional toss and let it simmer for about 15 minutes, or until the eggplant has softened but not turned mushy. Ingredients like rosemary, tomatoes, olives, and chickpeas would go well in this dish. Wait approximately 10 minutes, or until the beverage is at a comfortable temperature. Combine with a handful of parsley, minced. Some people like to top their stew with crumbled feta cheese.

Recipe : Greek Pasta

Prep Time : 0 Hour 15 Minutes

Total Time : 0 Hour 40 Minutes

Yields: 4 Servings

Material :

- A single 16-ounce package of penne noodles, a single spoonful of olive oil
  The equivalent of 1 milliliter of minced garlic.
- Tomatoes: 4 Roma (Plum) Tomatoes, diced
- 1 minced tiny
- 1.14-ounce (after draining) can of drained fava beans
- Chopped and put aside: 1 medium onion
- one-quarter cup lemon juice
- Half a cup of grated halloumi cheese.
- Twenty-five almond slices, or about a quarter cup

Step :

- Put on the stove top a large pot of water that has been lightly seasoned. After the pasta has been added, the water should be brought back to a boil. After 11 minutes, when the pasta is cooked through but still has a bite to it, whisk in the olive oil and garlic and continue cooking. Then, after the heat is at a medium-low setting, add the pasta back in.

- Toss the spaghetti with the tomatoes, pepper, fava beans, onion, and lemon juice. The pasta should be hot and the flavors incorporated after 7–8 minutes of cooking time. Garnish each serving with sliced almonds and halloumi cheese just before serving.

Recipe : Pesto-and-olive rolls

Prep Time : 0 Hour 55 Minutes

Total Time : 01 Hour 10 Minutes

Yields: 5 Servings

Material :

- 1 loaf of bread dough from the freezer, thawed to room temperature 13 c. BUITONI® Refrigerated Pesto with Basil and 1/2 c. BUITONI® Refrigerated Freshly Shredded Parmesan Cheese
- A couple of teaspoons of chopped kalamata olives (pitted, of course)
- 1.one large egg, beaten

Step :

- Roll out the dough into a 12-by-10-inch rectangle on a lightly floured board. Cover the dough with pesto, stopping half an inch from the edges. Add toppings like cheese and olives. Roll the dough into a cylinder that is 12 inches long, starting at the long end; pinch the ends to seal. Cut into 12 pieces, each approximately an inch long, and spread out on an unoiled baking sheet.

- Put it in a warm place, cover it with a damp cloth, and let it alone for 45 to 60 minutes, or until it has doubled in size. The rolls should be painted with beaten egg.
Raise the oven's heat to 350 degrees F.
Rolls should be baked for 20–25 minutes, until the tops are lightly browned and a hollow sound is produced when tapped on the bottom.

Recipe : Slump in the Mediterranean

Prep Time : 0 Hour 20 Minutes

Total Time : 01 Hour 20 Minutes

Yields: 12 Servings

Material :

- 8 ounces of softened cream cheese from an 8-ounce container
  One tablespoon of fresh lemon juice and three chopped garlic cloves.
- 1/2 milliliter of garlic powder 1 milligram of onion powder 1 teaspoon of Italian spice.
- One and a quarter cups of hummus.
- Roma tomatoes, seeded and diced (1 cup)
- Cucumbers, 1 cup, cut very small
- 1/2 cup kalamata olives, sliced
- 13 cups chopped red onion
- A dozen cups of crumbled feta

Step :

- In a mixing dish, stir together the thawed cream cheese, minced garlic, lemon juice, and Italian seasoning. In a circular dish with a diameter of approximately 10 inches, spread the mixture evenly over the bottom.
- Spread some hummus on top of it.Toss the tomatoes, cucumbers, olives, and red onion together in a bowl, and then top with hummus.

Then top with crumbled feta. To get the best flavor, let it chill in the fridge for at least an hour before serving.

Recipe : Mediterranean Eggplant Chicken

Prep Time : 0 Hour 50 Minutes

Total Time : 01 Hour 20 Minutes

Yields: 5   Servings

Material :

- One-half-inch thick slices of three peeled and sliced eggplants Three tablespoons of olive oil Six cubed chicken breast halves that have been deboned and skinned.
- An Onion, diced
- Tomato paste equaling 2 tablespoons
- a quarter cup liquid
- Amount: 2 teaspoons of dried oregano.
- to taste with salt and pepper.

Step :

- A half hour before you want to cook the eggplant, place the slices in a big saucepan with water that has been salted with a few tablespoons (this will improve the taste; they will leave a brown color in the pot).
- Once the eggplant has reached the desired doneness, remove it from the heat and brush it with olive oil. Transfer the meal to a 9-by-13-inch baking dish after a brief cook in a sauté pan or on the grill. Set Apart

- Place the chicken breasts and onion cubes in a large skillet and sauté over medium heat. After adding the tomato paste and water and giving everything a good stir, lower the heat to low, cover the pot, and let the mixture simmer for 10 minutes.
- Preheat the oven to 400 degrees Fahrenheit (200 degrees Celsius).
- The eggplant should be doused in the chicken and tomato sauce until it is well covered. Prepare the meal as usual, seasoning it with oregano, salt, and pepper, then wrap it in aluminum foil to keep it warm. Preparation time includes heating the oven to a high temperature and cooking for 20 minutes.

Recipe : Fish Soup

Prep Time : 0 Hour 10 Minutes

Total Time : 0 Hour 15 Minutes

Yields: 6 Servings

Material :

- Mix together 1 chopped onion, 1/2 chopped green bell pepper, and 2 minced garlic cloves. one chopped green bell pepper
- 1 14.5-ounce can drained chopped tomatoes
- 14 ounces of chicken broth spread among 2 cans
- 1 jar tomato paste or 1 jar tomato paste and 1 can tomato sauce (8 oz.)
- 2 cans of mushrooms, 2.25 oz. each
- Black olives, cut, a quarter cup
- Orange juice, half a cup
- A half-ounce of crisp white wine
- 2 bay leaves
- 1/4 of a fresh basil leaf
- About a quarter of a teaspoon of ground fennel seed
- ground black pepper equal to one-eighth of a teaspoon.
- Peeled and deveined medium-sized shrimp (one pound)
- One pound of cod fillets, frozen, defrosted, and cut into cubes.

Step :

- Put the onion, green bell pepper, garlic, tomatoes, chicken broth, tomato sauce, mushrooms, olives, orange juice, wine, bay leaves, dried basil, fennel seeds, and black pepper into a slow cooker and mix well. Cover and simmer on the lowest setting for four to four and a half hours, until the vegetables are crisp and tender.
- The shrimp and the cod should be combined. Cover. Shrimp should be cooked for 15–30 minutes, or until they become opaque. The bay leaves should be removed and discarded. Serve

Recipe : Med Pinwheels

Prep Time : 0 Hour 25 Minutes

Total Time : 0 Hour 45 Minutes

Yields: 20 Servings

Material :

- 1 container Pillsbury® crescent dinner rolls or 1 sheet Pillsbury® Crescent Recipe CreationsTM flaky doughTwelve pounds of cooked ham or prosciutto, sliced thin, four ounces of feta cheese, crumbled 1 can refrigerated flaky dough sheet Pillsbury®
- 1 and 1/2 teaspoons pepper
- 1 teaspoon of oil, preferably olive
- Chopped and weighed fresh basil, equaling 6 teaspoons.

Step :

- Then bring the oven temperature up to 375 degrees F. Cookie sheets should be greased with cooking spray before use.
- If you're using crescent rolls, unroll the dough and separate it into 4 squares. To close the holes, apply strong pressure. Press or roll each one into a square measuring 8 by 5 inches. If working with a dough sheet, unroll it and then divide it into four equal rectangles. Each one has to be flattened or rolled into an 8-by-5-inch rectangle.

- Arrange Distribute four slices of prosciutto evenly across each square. A small bowl should be used to combine the cheese, pepper, and oil. Distribute the mixture evenly over the prosciutto in the squares. Garnish with some chopped fresh basil.
- Each rectangle is to be rolled up starting at one of the shorter sides, and then the long edges must be sealed. The rolls should be cut into five equal pieces using a knife with a serrated edge. Spread out on baking pans, cut side up.
- Wait 15–20 minutes, or until the top is golden brown, before serving. Take the cookies off the baking sheets. Serve immediately while the food is still hot.

Recipe : Tuna salad

Prep Time : 0 Hour 5 Minutes

Total Time : 0 Hour 35 Minutes

Yields: 2 Servings

Material :

- 1 can of tuna in water, drained, measuring 6 ounces.
  3 teaspoons mayonnaise
  Spreadable hummus: 2 tbsp. spreadable hummus
- 8 olives, diced, or more according to personal preference.
- 1 teaspoon of dried oregano, or more according to personal preference.
- To taste, salt and freshly ground black pepper.

Step :

- Using a fork and a suitable container, make tuna flakes. Mix it in with hummus, olives, and mayonnaise. Spice it up with oregano, salt, and pepper. When you've mixed everything together, put it in the fridge for about half an hour to let the flavors develop.

Recipe : Salad kale

Prep Time : 0 Hour 20 Minutes

Total Time : 0 Hour 55 Minutes

Yields: 8 Servings

Material :

- 2 ounces of water in drops
Prepare 1 cup of red quinoa, or more to your liking.
One pound of plum tomatoes, whole.
- a quarter pound of butter
- 6-inch pieces of very finely chopped garlic
- 1 finely minced tiny shallot
- Juice from 2 lemons.
- Finely grated Parmesan cheese to the tune of 12 cups
- 1/4 mug of olive oil.
- A couple of 15-ounce cans of chickpeas, drained and rinsed
- About 3.5 bunches of kale, leaves removed and kale coarsely chopped.
- You may add 1 chopped red pepper to your salad.
- canned artichoke hearts (6.5 ounces), drained; more or less to taste
- A dozen cups of crumbled feta

Step :

- The quinoa and water should be brought to a boil in a saucepan. For another 15 to 20 minutes, reduce the heat to medium-low, cover the pot, and simmer the quinoa until it is soft.
- Prepare yet another pot of hot water. After 5 minutes, add the tomatoes, reduce the heat to low, and simmer until the tomatoes are soft, perhaps another 5 minutes. Remove the pan from the burner.
- Begin by melting butter in a skillet over medium heat. Warm the butter and add the lemon juice, then add the garlic and shallot and cook for about five minutes, or until the veggies are soft. Get rid of the stove's heat source.
- In the bowl of a food processor, combine the tomatoes, garlic mixture, Parmesan cheese, and 1/4 cup of olive oil. Make a smooth paste by blending. You should blend for at least a minute and a half.
- You may mix the quinoa, chickpeas, kale, and bell pepper in a bowl. Cooked pasta is topped with tomato sauce, artichoke hearts, and feta cheese before being served.

Recipe : Mediterranean Tuna Salad

Prep Time : 0 Hour 15 Minutes

Total Time : 0 Hour 15 Minutes

Yields: 4   Servings

Material :

- 14 cups of finely chopped red onion 14 cups of chopped and measured fresh parsley 2 cans of chunk light tuna in water, each 5 ounces.
- 3.0 ounces of olive oil.
- 2 tsp. of pure, unfiltered lemon juice.
- 12 teaspoons of lemon gratings.
- The equivalent of a quarter teaspoon of salt.
- One-fourth of a teaspoon of ground black pepper.

Step :

- Mix the tuna, onion, and parsley in a medium bowl.
  Olive oil, lemon juice, lemon zest, salt, and pepper should be combined to make the dressing. Put it in the bowl with the tuna and mix it together.

Recipe : Pacific salmon

Prep Time : 0 Hour 10 Minutes

Total Time : 0 Hour 25 Minutes

Yields: 4 Servings

Material :

- half a cup olive oil
  1/4 cup balsamic vinegar
  Squeeze the equivalent of four whole garlic
  cloves
- Salmon fillets (four, three-ounce portions)
- 1 tablespoon fresh cilantro, finely chopped
- 1 tablespoon fresh basil, finely chopped
- In a bowl, combine the garlic, salt, and 1.5
  teaspoons.

Step :

- Olive oil and balsamic vinegar should be put in a
  small bowl and stirred until smooth. Spread the
  salmon fillets out on a shallow baking tray. Turn
  the fillets over once after coating them with
  garlic, vinegar, and oil. Season with garlic salt,
  then stir in fresh herbs such as chopped cilantro
  and basil. Let it sit in the marinade for 10
  minutes.
- The oven's broiler must be preheated before
  use.

- Broil the salmon for about 15 minutes, flipping once, or until browned on both sides and easily flaked with a fork, keeping it about 15 cm away from the heat source. The meat should be occasionally glazed with the pan sauce.

Recipe : Capellini tuna

Prep Time : 0 Hour 15 Minutes

Total Time : 0 Hour 25 Minutes

Yields: 6 Servings

Material :

- 1 lb. cappelllini pasta, 3 lemons (zested and juiced) Fourteen cups of pure olive oil
- One-half cup of grated Parmesan cheese.
- 2 tablespoons of minced fresh parsley.
- 2 garlic cloves, chopped or minced.
- 12.5 tsp. salt
- Crushed red pepper flakes: 1 sprinkling, more or less to taste.
- One 5-ounce can of tuna packed in oil.
- 1/2 pound (approximately 15.5 ounces) cannellini beans, drained and rinsed

Step :

- Bring a large pot of lightly salted water to a boil. Put water into the cooking vessel. Once boiling again, add the capeline and simmer for another four to five minutes over medium heat, or until the pasta is al dente.
- Squeeze the lemons and pour the juice into a big bowl, taking care to get rid of the seeds. We recommend starting with the olive oil and thoroughly incorporating it into the dish. The

following components should be blended until smooth: Crushed red pepper, salt, garlic, lemon zest, parsley, and Parmesan cheese. Prior to incorporation, flake the tuna and crumble any large chunks. Incorporating cannellini beans requires gentle folding.

- You may add cappelletti pasta to the tuna mixture after it has been drained. Toss the ingredients together and serve immediately.

Recipe : Elote of the Mediterranean

Prep Time : 0 Hour 10 Minutes

Total Time : 0 Hour 25 Minutes

Yields: 5 Servings

Material :

- 1 washed and drained can of unseasoned cornThere are 12 of the little lemons.
  1 teaspoon olive oil-flavored mayonnaise
- 2 teaspoons of Crema fresca, or Mexican crema
- Mediterranean-style feta cheese, 14 qts.
- One Kalamata olive, halved, or more to taste.
- You may add as many or as few fresh basil leaves as you want, cut finely.
- The equivalent of one tiny sprinkle of smoked paprika

Step :

- Raise the oven temperature to 400 degrees Fahrenheit (200 degrees C). Using aluminum foil to line a baking sheet is a must.
  Spread the corn out on a baking sheet. Put in the lemon, pulp side up.
- It should take around 15–20 minutes for the corn and lemon to color while roasting in a preheated oven. Put it into a bowl and serve.
- Half of the lemon juice should be poured over the maize and mixed together. Mayonnaise

should be placed in the bowl's exact center.
Spread some crema over the mayonnaise.
Crumble some feta cheese on top of the crema.
As a finishing touch, sprinkle over some olives
and fresh basil. Sprinkle paprika over top, then
add any remaining lemon juice.

Recipe : Eggplant Pasta

Prep Time : 0 Hour 35 Minutes

Total Time : 0 Hour 55 Minutes

Yields: 10 Servings

Material :

- 1 eggplant, cut to a thickness of 3/4 inch, a pinch of salt, and 9 ounces pappardelle pasta (wide fettuccine noodles)
- equivalent to three teaspoons olive oil
- One small onion, coarsely diced.
- Three minced garlic cloves (or one large bulb),
- Dry oregano, 2 teaspoons
- 1 can of crushed tomatoes (18-ounce capacity).
- Red wine vinegar, 1 table spoon.
- Just a pinch of salt, one teaspoon.
- A white sugar cube is equal to 1 mm3.
- Black pepper, freshly ground, 12 teaspoons.
- 12 pounds of diced fresh buffalo mozzarella cheese.
- 1/2 cup of fresh basil, freshly chopped, or more if desired.

Step :

- Sprinkle a little dusting of salt over the eggplant slices and place them in a colander. Ten minutes of draining time is recommended for the eggplant. In order to prepare eggplant for cooking, just wash it and pat it dry with paper towels. Separately, cut the eggplant into cubes.

- Start by bringing a large pot of lightly salted water to a boil. The ideal cooking time for pappardelle is 10 to 11 minutes in boiling water, at which point it will be tender but still have a little bite.
- 1.5 teaspoons, cooked on medium heatTo get a browned exterior, cook the eggplant for 5 to 10 minutes, turning regularly and adding extra oil if it dries up. The eggplant should be moved to a bowl while the oil is still in the pan.
- The remaining oil should be heated in the same pan, and the onion and garlic should be sautéed there until they are golden brown, which should take around 10 minutes of steady stirring. Return the eggplant to the pan, sprinkle with oregano, and cook for one more minute while stirring.
- Add some tomato sauce, vinegar, salt, and sugar to your eggplant mixture. Bring the sauce to a boil with the lid on for about 10 minutes, or until the eggplant has softened. Mix the pasta and sauce together in a bowl, then top with the mozzarella and basil.

Recipe : Greek Orange Salad

Prep Time : 0 Hour 20 Minutes

Total Time : 0 Hour 20 Minutes

Yields: 4 Servings

Material :

- I have four oranges.
  Three blood oranges
  One small onion, coarsely diced.
- 3.0 ounces of olive oil.
- Approximately 2 tablespoons lemon juice
- salt
- Totaling just 1 tiny, freshly ground peppercorn
- 1 ounce of black olives, dried

Step :

- Cut off the top and bottom of each orange to provide a flat cutting surface. Use a small, sharp knife to carefully remove the peel and pith from the fruit without taking off too much of the fruit itself. Oranges should be cut horizontally and then put in a decorative pattern on a serving platter.
- Put the oranges in a bowl and drizzle the mixture of onion, olive oil, lemon juice, and salt over them. Use freshly ground pepper and finish off the salad by scattering the black olives on top.

Recipe : Orzo salad

Prep Time : 0 Hour 20 Minutes

Total Time : 0 Hour 55 Minutes

Yields: 6   Servings

Material :

- Half of a 16-ounce package of uncooked orzo There should be 12 pounds of cherry tomatoes and 12 cups of chopped red onion.
- One Cup of Cucumber, diced
- One cup of pitted and halved Mediterranean olives.
- A cup of chopped Asiago cheese amounts to 1 cup.

Step :

- Start by bringing a large pot of lightly salted water to a boil. To prepare orzo, bring a pot of water to a boil and add salt. Cook the orzo for about 9 minutes, turning occasionally, until it is al dente. Make sure to drain properly. After washing with cold water, drain the liquid well once more.
- Mix the orzo, cherry tomatoes, red onion, cucumber, olives, and Asiago cheese in a large bowl.
- To make the vinaigrette, mix the garlic, olive oil, red wine vinegar, lemon juice, salt, and pepper in a small bowl and whisk together. Drizzle over

the orzo mixture and stir lightly to combine. Once you've added the basil and parsley, mix thoroughly. Stir occasionally and let the flavors combine for 20 minutes.

Recipe : Stuffed Zucchini

Prep Time : 0 Hour 20 Minutes

Total Time : 01 Hour 20 Minutes

Yields: 4 Servings

Material :

- Zoodles: 1 big zucchini, halved lengthwise.
  2 teaspoons butter
  1 medium sliced sweet onion
- The minced equivalent of one tablespoon of garlic,
- 1.05 kg ground lamb
- flavored with coarse salt.
- Grind the black peppercorns to the desired consistency.
- The contents of one (16-ounce) can of tomato sauce
- In a small bowl, combine 2 tomato slices.
- Crumbled feta cheese equaling a quarter cup
- 1/2 teaspoon pine nuts
- 1/8 teaspoon of mint
- 1/3 cup of liquid.
- A quarter of a cup of mint leaves
- About 3/4 cup of bread crumbs with seasonings
- 1/4 cup of mozzarella cheese, shredded

Step :

- Turn the oven temperature up to 450 degrees F. (230 degrees C).
- Carve out each half of the zucchini while leaving a shell that is about half an inch thick, and then separate and remove the pulp and seeds from the zucchini using a melon baller. Reduce the pulp of the zucchini to pieces that are around 14 inches in diameter. Discard seeds.
- Heat olive oil in a large pan over medium heat. To soften the onion and garlic, cook them in heated oil while stirring occasionally for approximately five minutes. Add the ground lamb, and continue to boil while stirring for 5 to 7 minutes, or until the meat is gently browned. Combine the lamb with the zucchini that has been diced. Turn the temperature down to medium-low. Simmer the mixture for approximately three minutes, or until the zucchini is at the desired temperature. Get rid of any extra oil. Add coarse salt and black pepper to the ground lamb mixture, and mix well.
- Turn off the heat in the skillet.After combining the lamb mixture with the tomato sauce, tomatoes, feta cheese, pine nuts, and a quarter cup of chopped mint leaves, pour the mixture into the halves of zucchini. Place the filled zucchini halves in an oven-safe dish of sufficient size. The baking dish needs some water, so pour some in there.
- Bake for half an hour in an oven that has been preheated. In a bowl, combine the bread crumbs and the mozzarella cheese. On top of the zucchini, sprinkle a quarter cup's worth of mint

leaves, then cover with the bread crumbs mixture. Continue baking for about another ten minutes, or until the top is crispy and browned.

Recipe : Mediterranean Veggies

Prep Time : 0 Hour 20 Minutes

Total Time : 0 Hour 30 Minutes

Yields: 3   Servings

Material :

- 2 teaspoons butter
  Onions, chopped; 12 cups The equivalent of 2 cups of sliced carrots,
- One green bell pepper, diced.
- One red bell pepper, cut into little cubes.
- 1 fennel bulb, thinly sliced
- Dried Italian herb mix, 2 tablespoons minimum, more to taste.
- To taste, with salt and freshly ground black pepper.

Step :

- In a large pan, heat the olive oil and sauté the onion over medium heat for approximately 5 minutes, or until it is transparent and has softened. After adding the carrots, bell peppers, and fennel, continue cooking while stirring regularly for 5 to 10 minutes, or until the vegetables have become tender but are still somewhat chewy. Add some Italian herbs, salt, and pepper before serving.

Recipe : Mediterranean Cauliflower

Prep Time : 0 Hour 15 Minutes

Total Time : 0 Hour 30 Minutes

Yields: 4 Servings

Material :

- 1 tablespoon olive oil
  Lime juice, 1.5 mL
  1 teaspoon dried oregano
- 0.5 gram salt
- 1/8 teaspoon ground black pepper
- 1 small cauliflower head, cut into florets and chunks
- 1/4 cup Athenos® brand crumbled feta cheese, with a Mediterranean flavor profile,

Step :

- Set the temperature of an air fryer to 375 degrees Fahrenheit (190 degrees Celsius).
- Olive oil, lemon juice, oregano, salt, and pepper should be mixed together in a small bowl and whisked.
- Place the cauliflower florets in a large resealable bag. Lightly shake the container after drizzling the coating over the oil mixture to disperse it evenly. Place the cauliflower florets in a single layer in the air fryer's basket. Work in shifts as required.

- Air-fry the cauliflower for 12–15 minutes, shaking the basket every 4–5 minutes, until golden and crispy. Stir the feta cheese into the hot cauliflower in the serving dish.

Recipe : Branzino

Prep Time : 0 Hour 15 Minutes

Total Time : 0 Hour 40 Minutes

Yields: 4   Servings

Material :

- Combine 1 red onion, 1 tablespoon of olive oil, salt and pepper to taste, and a chop of both.
- Two cleaned whole branzino (sea bass).
- There are four halved lemon slices.
- Dried and fresh rosemary equal two sprigs.
- 1/4 of an ounce of dry white
- 1 tablespoon lemon juice
- 1 tablespoon of fresh oregano leaves
- 14 cups of chopped Italian flat-leafed parsley

Step :

- The oven has to be heated to 325 degrees F. (165 degrees C).
  Add some red onion to a large baking dish, season with salt and pepper, and sprinkle with 1 tablespoon of olive oil.
- The baking dish should include two whole fish, heads and tails included. In each opening, place a slice of lemon, a sprig of rosemary, and a little amount of the red onion from the pan. After the fish has been marinated in white wine and

lemon juice, sprinkle it with oregano. Use the remaining olive oil to sprinkle over the fish.

- Twenty-five minutes after preheating the oven, check to see whether the fish is opaque and flakes easily with a fork.
- Carefully push a spatula through the gaps, then remove the bones to reveal the fish. Decorate the fish with two slices of lemon and some chopped parsley and serve.

Recipe : Meatballs

Prep Time : 0 Hour 30 Minutes

Total Time : 01 Hour 10 Minutes

Yields: 8 Servings

Material :

- Two pounds of lean ground beef (fat content of 90% or less)
  1 large egg whisked with 1/3 cup dry bread crumbsThe equivalent of one tablespoon of butter.
- 1/3 cup minced onion
- 2 garlic cloves, minced or chopped
- 1 tbsp of minced fresh rosemary leaves equals
- 14 cups of parsley, fresh, minced.
- 1/2 teaspoon of dried oregano and 1 tablespoon of fresh, chopped oregano
- 1 tablespoon fresh dill, finely chopped
- 1 teaspoon of freshly ground coriander.
- Kosher salt, about 1.5 teaspoons (more or less to taste).
- Add as much or as little freshly ground black pepper as desired.
- Cooking pans should be sprayed with olive oil.
- (Optional)

Step :

- Start by preheating the oven to 375 degrees Fahrenheit (190 degrees Celsius). Get ready for the recipe by preparing a sheet pan with foil or parchment paper.
  Combine the ground beef, egg, bread crumbs, onion, garlic, rosemary, parsley, oregano, dill, and coriander with the salt and pepper in a large mixing basin. Use your hands to thoroughly blend the ingredients.
- Form the beef mixture into 1-inch-diameter balls and place them on the prepared baking sheet.
- For about 40 minutes, or until the meatballs are browned and the center is no longer pink, coat them with cooking spray and bake them in a preheated oven.
- The meatballs are done when they can be removed from the oven and placed on a dish lined with paper towels to cool for a short while. Extra chopped fresh parsley should be used as a garnish before serving.

Recipe : Skillet-cooked Mediterranean chicken

Prep Time : 0 Hour 10 Minutes

Total Time : 0 Hour 25 Minutes

Yields: 4 Servings

Material :

- Oregano, dry, one-half a teaspoon 12 teaspoon black pepperThe equivalent of a pinch of salt
- These are four skinless, boneless chicken breast halves. Total weight: 6 ounces.
- One olive oil tablespoon, cut in half.
- Cut 1 small lemon into 8 wedges.
- Fill a 14-ounce jar with 8 ounces of sun-dried tomatoes, packed in oil and drained.
- 2 medium-sized garlic cloves, chopped
- 1 package (8.8 oz.) Uncle Ben's® Ready Rice® Roasted Chicken Flavored Rice is included.
- Approximately 1/3 cup of unsalted chicken stock.
- Baby spinach, fresh, around 6 ounces for one bag.
- 1 ounce of feta cheese crumbles, 1 gram (optional).
- 2-tablespoons of roasted pine nuts

Step :

- Half a teaspoon of oregano, a quarter of a teaspoon of black pepper, and salt to taste. distributed uniformly over the bird's skin.
- In a skillet with a 10-inch diameter, heat 1 tablespoon of oil over medium heat. Chicken, seasoned side down, should be added to the pan. Keep the cover on for about six minutes, or until the meat is browned. After you turn the chicken over, lay two lemon slices on top of each breast. The internal temperature of the chicken should reach 165 degrees Fahrenheit, so cover and continue cooking for another 6 minutes. Keep the chicken warm by placing it on a dish and covering it haphazardly with foil.
- Keep the same pan and heat the extra tablespoon of oil over medium heat. While stirring frequently, continue cooking for another minute after adding the garlic and sun-dried tomatoes. Add the rice, the remaining chicken stock, the remaining 1/2 teaspoon of oregano, and the remaining 1/4 teaspoon of pepper to a saucepan and mix well. Wilt the spinach by adding it in tiny amounts and stirring it slowly. Return the chicken breasts to the pan. Add some cheese and pine nuts for garnish.

Recipe : Navy bean stew

Prep Time : 0 Hour 15 Minutes

Total Time : 01 Hour 0 Minutes

Yields: 6   Servings

Material :

- 3.0 ounces of olive oil.
  1 medium diced onion
  1 medium-sized diced tomato
- 1 medium-sized chopped red pepper
- Very coarsely chop 3 whole garlic cloves.
- There are four new sage leaves in this.
- 1 fresh sprig of rosemary.
- pepper to taste, at least a quarter of a teaspoon of crushed red pepper
- To taste, with salt and freshly ground black pepper.
- Three 16-ounce cans of washed, drained, and cooked navy beans.
- One bay leaf
- Add 3 cups of water, or just enough to cover the contents.
- Finely chopped fresh chives, at least 2 tablespoons and more to taste.

Step :

- Oil should be heated over medium heat in a skillet before the onion is added. About five minutes of cooking time, with regular stirring, should be enough for the onion to soften and become translucent. Add the tomato and bell pepper after about three minutes of boiling and keep on simmering until the pepper is soft. Keep heating and stirring for another minute or so after adding the garlic to allow the scent to fully develop. Season with salt, pepper, red pepper flakes, sage, and rosemary, and stir to combine. Reduce the heat to low and continue to cook for another 5 minutes.

- Heat the bean mixture and bay leaf in a large saucepan over medium. Put the vegetable mix in the saucepan. Put in sufficient water to completely submerge it. The beans should be cooked for about half an hour, stirred occasionally, and given a little additional water if they seem to be drying out.
- Do not wait to serve after topping with chives.

Recipe : Chopped Kale from the Mediterranean

Prep Time : 0 Hour 15 Minutes

Total Time : 0 Hour 25 Minutes

Yields: 6 Servings

Material :

- One dozen cups of chopped kale.
  Juice of half a lemon, about 2
  tablespoons.Add olive oil to taste (about 1
  teaspoon).
- The equivalent of one tablespoon of minced
  garlic.
- Soy sauce, 0.1 milliliter
- The perfect amount of salt
- Grind the black peppercorns to the desired
  consistency.

Step :

- Fill a saucepan with water until it reaches a
  level just below the steamer's base, then insert
  the steamer. To get the water boiling, cover the
  pot and set it over high heat. Cover the
  saucepan after adding the kale and steam it for
  seven to ten minutes, adjusting the time based
  on the kale's thickness.

- To make the dressing, mix together the lemon
  juice, olive oil, garlic, soy sauce, salt, and pepper

in a large bowl. Steamed kale may be added to the dressing and tossed until it is evenly coated.

Recipe : Tilapia

Prep Time : 0 Hour 15 Minutes

Total Time : 0 Hour 25 Minutes

Yields: 4 Servings

Material :

- Two tilapia fillets, three sun-dried tomatoes packed in oil, drained and chopped, and one tablespoon of drained capers,
- 1 tsp. of the oil from the sun-dried tomato jar
- Lime juice, 1.5 mL
- Chop kalamata olives into 2 teaspoons.

Step :

- Start by preheating the oven to 375 degrees Fahrenheit (190 degrees Celsius). In a small bowl, combine the sun-dried tomatoes, olives, and capers and stir to combine. Put it off to the side.
- The tilapia fillets should be laid out in a baking dish so that they are parallel to one another. After sprinkling with oil, add a splash of lemon juice.

- Fish should flake readily when checked with a fork after being baked for 10–15 minutes in a preheated oven. Overcooking the fish might lead to it being dry, so check on it after 10 minutes. Serve the fish over a bed of tomato sauce when cooking is complete.

Recipe : Chickpea stew

Prep Time : 0 Hour 20 Minutes

Total Time : 0 Hour 50 Minutes

Yields: 4 Servings

Material :

- one-quarter cup virgin olive oil
  One large, chopped red onion One Italian
  parsley bunch, chopped.
- 2 garlic cloves, minced or chopped
- One little carrot, coarsely shredded.
- 1 medium-sized diced eggplant
- 2 cups of chickpeas, cooked and rinsed with the
  excess sodium removed.
- Cherry tomatoes (one cup) halved lengthwise
- Vegetable broth, about 12 cups (more if you
  want).
- 1/4 teaspoon of dried oregano
- 1 teaspoon of dried thyme.
- One dozen pepper flakes with a teaspoon of red
  pepper
- Sprinkle with salt and freshly ground black
  pepper to taste.

Step :

- A Dutch oven placed over medium heat is ideal
  for warming olive oil. Sauté the onion in the hot
  oil for about 5 minutes, or until it is soft and

transparent. Parsley and garlic should be cooked for two minutes with steady stirring. Mix it up often for the next minute or two after you add the shredded carrot. The eggplant should be sautéed for two or three minutes after being added to the pan.

- Incorporate the canned tomatoes and chickpeas into the cooking mixture. Add in some oregano, thyme, and cayenne pepper, too. Bring everything to a full boil together. Put the stew over low heat and let it cook for about 15 minutes, or until the vegetables are soft and the stew has thickened. Toss in some more broth if you feel it's necessary. To taste, sprinkle a little salt and pepper on the food just before serving.

Recipe : Empanadas

Prep Time : 0 Hour 35 Minutes

Total Time : 0 1 Hour 25 Minutes

Yields: 6   Servings

Material :

- 1 1/2 skinless, boneless chicken breasts4 whole garlic cloves, peeled, chopped, and halved.
- You'll need between 1 and 14 tablespoons of balsamic vinegar, divided equally.
- One dozen dried teaspoons of oregano.
- Sprinkle with salt and freshly ground black pepper to taste.
- The equivalent of one cup of chopped tomatoes was
- Onion, minced finely, 1/2 cup.
- One lemon's juice

Step :

- Chicken strips, 2 tbsp olive oil, 2 tbsp minced garlic, 1 tsp balsamic vinegar, 1 tsp dried oregano, salt, and pepper should be combined in a bowl. Allow 30 minutes for marinating.
- Tomatoes and onions should be combined with the remaining tablespoon of olive oil, two minced garlic cloves, and a quarter of a teaspoon of balsamic vinegar. Just before serving, season with a pinch of salt and pepper.

Hold off on eating for 30 minutes as the flavors combine.

- Raise the oven temperature to 400 degrees Fahrenheit (200 degrees Celsius). Heat a pan over medium heat and sear the chicken for about five to eight minutes, or until the juices run clear. In a skillet, shred the chicken using two forks to get bite-sized chunks. Add the juice of half a lemon to the pan as a final step in the cooking process.
- Cut the dough in half to make six individual pizzas. Roll each piece into a 6-inch circle on a floured board, folding in the fresh basil as you go.
- Spinach, chicken, mozzarella, and tomato sauce should be layered on one side of each circle. Once the dough has been folded over the filling, the curved edge should be pressed to seal the fold.
- It's best to use a light coating of olive oil to grease a baking sheet. Before placing the empanadas on the baking sheet, lightly brush the tops with olive oil.
- Toast the topping in a preheated oven for 12–15 minutes, or until it reaches the desired color.

Recipe : Mediterranean Clams

Prep Time : 0 Hour 15 Minutes

Total Time : 0 Hour 25 Minutes

Yields: 6 Servings

Material :

- Bread crumbs (1 cup) and pine nuts (1/2 tablespoon)
  Two minced or sliced garlic cloves,
- Prepped littleneck clams weigh 3 pounds.
- Diced fresh basil equals 1/4 cup.
- 1 tablespoon melted butter
- 1/2 cup halved cherry tomatoes

Step :

- The temperature in the oven should be raised to 350 degrees Fahrenheit (175 degrees Celsius). On a baking sheet, mix together the pine nuts, garlic, and bread crumbs.
  It should take around 5 minutes to toast in an oven that has been preheated, and the process should be continued until the bread is just browned.
- In the meantime, a saucepan should have a steamer insert put inside of it, and then the saucepan should be filled with water until it reaches a position that is just below the bottom of the steamer. This will allow the food to be steamed. Bring the water to the point where it is

rapidly boiling. Once the clams have been added, cover the saucepan and steam them for around five minutes, or until their shells have opened.

- After the bread crumbs have been toasted, put them in a big bowl along with the other ingredients. After adding the tomatoes and basil, thoroughly combine all of the ingredients. When you are ready to serve the clams, briefly toss them in the mixture of bread crumbs and butter.

Recipe : Mediterranean Chicken with Vegetables

Prep Time : 0 Hour 30 Minutes

Total Time : 06 Hour 25 Minutes

Yields: 8 Servings

Material :

- Ground coriander equals one teaspoon. Seasoning: 1 teaspoon salt, 1/4 teaspoon ground cumin.
- The equivalent of one-fourth of a teaspoon of cayenne pepper
- Eight bone-in, skinless chicken thighs.
- a 15-ounce can of rinsed and drained chickpeas
- One 14-ounce can of chopped tomatoes, unsalted and unopened.
- A dozen artichoke hearts, marinated and drained
- Diced large carrots (4.25 g)
- Split four large garlic cloves in half.
- The equivalent of one cinnamon stick, three inches in length,
- 1 teaspoon of olive oil, or more to taste.
- One large, sweet onion, halved lengthwise and then thinly sliced.
- Green beans, 12 lbs., washed and halved lengthwise
- Pepper, red, one, peeled, seeded, and sliced into 1-inch chunks.
- Cilantro, cut coarsely, 14 cups

- approximately 3 liters of water
- Mix 2 cups of couscous with 2 cups of water.

Step :

- Place the spices (turmeric, ginger, coriander, cumin, and cayenne pepper) in a small cup. For best results, apply the mixture to the chicken and let it sit for at least half an hour.
Combine the chickpeas, chopped tomatoes, artichoke hearts, carrots, garlic, and cinnamon stick in the bottom of a slow cooker that is between 6 and 7 quarts in size.
To heat the olive oil, use a big, nonstick skillet and bring it to medium heat. Put in the chicken and cook for four minutes on each side, or until browned. Chicken with the bone side up should be placed in the slow cooker. Throw the chopped onion into the same pan. The onions should be sautéed for about five minutes over medium heat, or until they have become a golden yellow hue and have developed brown edges thanks to the addition of turmeric. Toss it into the slow cooker and turn the heat to low.
- Cover the slow cooker, set the temperature to low, and simmer for two hours.
- Arrange the green beans and bell pepper on top of the chicken. Keep on simmering for another two to three hours with the lid on.
- Meanwhile, start boiling three cups of water. After adding the couscous, stir it up to ensure even distribution. Turn off the stove and take the cover off the saucepan. Sit back and relax for

5–10 minutes as the water is absorbed and the couscous softens.

- Start by spreading some warm couscous on each plate, and then add layers of chicken and vegetables. Transfer some of the liquid from the slow cooker to serve with each serving.

Recipe : Agnolotti mushrooms

Prep Time : 0 Hour 10 Minutes

Total Time : 0 Hour 16 Minutes

Yields: 3   Servings

Material :

- 1 package (nine ounces) BUITONI® Riserva Refrigerated All Natural Wild Mushroom Agnolotti
  A quarter of a bunch of fresh sage 3 tablespoons of olive oil.
- Black pepper, ground to a fine powder, 1 particle.
- 1/4 cup BUITONI® Freshly Shredded Parmesan Cheese

Step :

- Bring the water to a boil in a big pot. Add the pasta when the water boils and cook for four minutes. Over medium heat, bring a big saucepan's worth of oil to a low simmer. The temperature should be reduced after putting in the sage leaves. Keep cooking for another minute and a half, or until the leaves have shrunk and turned crisp. Take off the leaves of sage from the pan.
- The pasta should be drained after 4 minutes, and 1/4 cup of the cooking water should be reserved. Put the saved cooking water back into

the pan. Return the drained pasta to the pan and cook for another 30 seconds over medium heat, or until some of the water has been absorbed. Sprinkle some pepper on top, and then cover everything with cheese and the sage leaves you saved. When it's done cooking, serve immediately.

Prep Time : 0 Hour 35 Minutes

Total Time : 01 Hour 50 Minutes

Yields: 6 Servings

Material :

- a single teaspoon of Marie's® Coleslaw Dressing, OriginalSeason with paprika 12 tsp. of cumin
- Cinnamon, one-eighth of a teaspoon
- Three whole garlic cloves, minced.
- Optional (Optional) (Optional)
- zest and juice from one lemon.
- 1/2 teaspoon salt
- equivalent to 12 teaspoons ground black pepper
- Cut up four boneless chicken breasts into bite-sized pieces.
- In a bowl, add 1 large onion that has been finely sliced.
- Eight wet wooden skewers
- shredded green cabbage, equivalent to half a cabbage head,
- 12 extremely thin slices of red onion
- Chop 1 small bunch of flat-leaf parsley and set aside.
- Dressing required to make 1/2 cup Marie's® Original Coleslaw
- Optional (Optional) (Optional)

Step :

- Put all of the following into a dish and stir to combine; this is the marinade for the chicken. The recipe includes Marie's Original Coleslaw Dressing, a variety of spices (including paprika, cumin, cinnamon, garlic, red pepper flakes), fresh lemon, lemon zest, fresh lemon juice, salt, and pepper. Be sure to give it a good whisk until everything is evenly incorporated.
- Arrange alternate chicken and onion pieces on each skewer and lay them in a shallow baking dish. Leave the chicken skewers in the marinade for a while to absorb the flavor before setting them aside. Cover and place in the fridge for at least an hour and no more than a day to chill.
- Mix the cabbage, onion, and parsley in a large basin for the slaw. Mix in Marie's Original Coleslaw Dressing. Red pepper flakes may be sprinkled on top of the meal just before serving for extra heat.
- Get a medium-high fire going in the grill. Grill marinated chicken skewers after coating the grill rack with oil. Turn the skewers every few minutes once the chicken has cooked for around 15 minutes. Serve immediately with Marie's Original Coleslaw Dressing on the side and a side of warm pita bread, sliced tomatoes, slaw, and more dressing.

Recipe : Mediterranean Chicken Kabobs

Prep Time : 0 Hour 20 Minutes

Total Time : 04 Hour 40 Minutes

Yields: 6   Servings

Material :

- Six boneless, skinless chicken breast halves, lightly seasoned
  8 large garlic cloves, diced; additional garlic cloves may be added to taste.
- 1/2 cup olive oil
- Two teaspoons of apple cider vinegar, more if desired.
- A splash (or more) of red wine vinegar, at least 2 teaspoons.
- White balsamic vinegar, about 2 teaspoons (more if desired).
- 2 tablespoons fresh lemon juice, plus more to taste
- Red pepper flakes, about 1 tablespoon.
- 1 teaspoon ground allspice
- Sumac powder, one tablespoon
- 1/8 of a teaspoon of pomegranate syrup

Step :

- Make sure you salt the chicken breasts before you cook them. From each breast, you should have three to four servings. Combine all the

ingredients in a big bowl and stir in the garlic.
Put in the dish some olive oil, some apple cider
vinegar, some red wine vinegar, some white
balsamic vinegar, some lemon juice, some red
pepper flakes, some allspice, some sumac, and
some pomegranate syrup. Use your hands to stir
and blend gently.

- The chicken mixture should be wrapped in
  plastic wrap and pushed down to remove any
  pockets of air. Put it in the fridge for at least
  four hours and up to a full day.
  It is best to close the lid and heat an outdoor
  grill with two grill baskets for ten minutes.
  Distribute the chicken among the grill baskets
  so that each gets about the same amount. 10–15
  minutes on the grill each side for medium-rare
  to well-done meat.

Recipe : Farfalle from the Mediterranean

Prep Time : 0 Hour 10 Minutes

Total Time : 0 Hour 15 Minutes

Yields: 3 Servings

Material :

- There should be 1 box of farfalle pasta (containing 12 ounces).
  1 pound chorizo sausage, shredded14 cups of fresh basil, cut into ribbons.
- 1 pound crumbled chorizo
- 1/2 cups of pine nuts
- Two minced or chopped garlic cloves.
- One-half cup of grated Parmesan cheese.
- a single cup diced tomatoes
- 1/2 cup olive oil
- To make red wine vinegar, you'll need 14 cups.

Step :

- Salted water brought to a boil is ideal for cooking pasta.
- While the pasta is boiling, brown the chorizo in a pan. Toss in the nuts and toast them, watching closely so they don't burn. Stop the cooking process after the garlic has been added.
- Prepare a colander to collect the drained pasta. In a large bowl, stir together the pasta, chorizo mixture, basil, cheese, and tomatoes. Toss

together the spaghetti with the olive oil and balsamic vinegar, then pour over the spaghetti and toss to coat. Serve

Recipe : One-Pot Chicken Mediterranean

Prep Time : 0 Hour 15 Minutes

Total Time : 0 Hour 45 Minutes

Yields: 6 Servings

Material :

- a single stick of butter
  12 cups of chopped onions
  1 minced garlic clove
- An Italian spice dose of 1 mg per teaspoon?
- 1 teaspoon dried basil
- seasoned with salt.
- Two 14-ounce cans of artichoke hearts, drained and quartered
- Crushed tomatoes fill one 28-ounce can.
- One can of chopped tomatoes (14.5 ounces total).
- 6 ounces of black olives from a can, cut in half.
- 1 4.5-ounce can of sliced mushrooms, drained
- There are four boneless, skinless chicken breasts in this dish.

Step :

- Butter has to be melted in a big pan over medium heat. Salt, onions, garlic, Italian seasoning, and basil are all good additions to this. It has to be sautéed for around five minutes, or until it develops a golden brown color.

- Cook until boiling, then add in the artichoke hearts, crushed tomatoes, diced tomatoes, olives, and mushrooms. Cover the pan after the chicken has been added and reduce the heat to medium. Toss the mixture occasionally and simmer for 20–25 minutes, or until the chicken is well cooked and the juices flow clear.

Recipe : Mediterranean Chicken Breast

Prep Time : 0 Hour 10 Minutes

Total Time : 01 Hour 0 Minutes

Yields: 2 Servings

Material :

- Two eight-ounce chicken breasts without the bone or skin, freshly ground black pepper, kosher salt, and a quarter cup of olive oil.
- 1/4 cup of lemon juice, squeezed
- One minced garlic clove.
- Half a teaspoon of dried oregano, or more to taste.
- Thyme, dried, 1/4 teaspoon (or more to taste).

Step :

- Season the chicken breasts on both sides with salt and pepper and place them in a covered dish or container. Chicken breasts should be marinated in a combination of olive oil, lemon juice, garlic, oregano, and thyme. Keep the meat at room temperature for 10 minutes during marinating.
- Prepare for an oven temperature of 400 degrees Fahrenheit (200 degrees C). Put a baking sheet on a rack that's approximately 6 inches from the oven's broiler.

- Spread the chicken breasts out in a baking dish and pour the marinade over them.
- Pre-heat the oven to 350 degrees Fahrenheit and place the chicken on the middle rack. Bake the chicken until it is no longer pink in the center and the juices run clear, about 35 to 45 minutes. Place the baking dish on the oven's highest rack and broil the chicken for 5 minutes, or until it is evenly browned.

Recipe : Frittata Mediterranean

Prep Time : 0 Hour 20 Minutes

Total Time : 0 Hour 45 Minutes

Yields: 8   Servings

Material :

- 1 (12-ounce) package of chicken sausage, sliced into 1/2-inch-thick rounds
  1 1/2 cups finely chopped zucchini
  1 cup of halved grape tomatoes
- One pound of red onions, peeled, cut, and chopped
- A spoonful of olive oil
- Twelve large eggs
- 1.25 ounces of milk
- a quarter of a teaspoon of kosher salt
- There is ground black pepper equal to 12 teaspoons.
- 1/4 cup crumbled feta cheese
- One tablespoon of fresh dill, chopped.

Step :

- Turn the temperature in the oven up to 400 degrees F. (200 degrees C). (200 degrees C).
- Spread the sausage, zucchini, grape tomatoes, and red onion evenly on a rimmed baking sheet. It's best to add the olive oil after the ingredients have already been combined. Create a single

layer by spreading
Roast in an oven that has been preheated until
the edges are browned, which should take
roughly seven minutes.

- Take the sausage mixture out of the oven, and
  then decrease the temperature to 375 degrees
  Fahrenheit (190 degrees Celsius) (190 degrees
  Celsius).
- In a bowl, whisk together the eggs, milk, salt,
  and pepper. After everything has been placed
  equally, sprinkle feta cheese all over the top of
  the sausage mixture.
- Place the baking sheet back in the oven and
  continue baking for 17 to 20 minutes, or until
  the eggs have set.
- Sprinkle some dill on top after serving.

Recipe : Mediterranean Couscous Salad

Prep Time : 0 Hour 15 Minutes

Total Time : 01 Hour 5 Minutes

Yields: 4   Servings

Material :

- Olive oil, to taste, 2 teaspoons
  Couscous, 2 servings
  Approximately half a cup dried mung beans
- Four quarts of vegetable stock.
- The equivalent of 2 tablespoons of salt, split
- Diced Cucumber (One)
- 2 tomatoes, diced
- A squeezed lemon's worth
- Chopped cilantro equals 1 tbsp.
- There is ground black pepper equal to 12
  teaspoons.

Step :

- Before adding the ingredients, start a multi-
  functional pressure cooker (such as an Instant
  Pot®) on the Saute setting.Olive oil should be
  heated before being combined with couscous
  and mung beans. Keep stirring for the whole
  two minutes of cooking time. Add in the
  vegetable broth and the teaspoon of salt. Just
  reattach it and again check the lock. Choose high
  pressure as directed by the manufacturer and

set the timer for twenty minutes. Let the pressure build up for around ten to fifteen minutes.

- Follow the manufacturer's directions for ten minutes of natural pressure release, and then utilize the quick-release method for the remaining pressure for five minutes. The cover may be accessed by turning the key and uncovering the device. The couscous has to be fluffed with a fork before it can be served. Wait around 10 minutes for the temperature to drop.
- In a dish, stir together the couscous, mung beans, cucumber, tomatoes, lemon juice, and cilantro. Use a pinch of salt and a pinch of pepper per serving, or to taste.

Recipe : Mediterranean Made Rights

Prep Time : 0 Hour 20 Minutes

Total Time : 01 Hour 0 Minutes

Yields: 6 Servings

Material :

- Olive oil, to taste, 2 teaspoons
  Approximately 1 pound of ground lamb Minced
  onions, up to 12 cups
- One milligram of finely chopped lemon rind.
- Dry oregano, equivalent to 12 teaspoons
- One-half of a teaspoon of minced dried garlic
- 1 and 1/2 teaspoons salt
- 1/2 milligram ground black pepper
- 1/3 cup lime juice
- 1 oz. liquid
- standard yogurt (6 ounce) carton
- Cheese, feta, crumbled, 3 ounces
- A pinch of dried oregano, or a quarter teaspoon
- a little less than a teaspoon garlic powder
- a pinch of lemon zest
- to taste, with salt and pepper.
- Six pita breads were cut into discs.

Step :

- Olive oil should be heated in a large pan over
  moderate heat. Lamb should be cooked until it
  begins to come apart after being stirred in.

When you add the onions, you need to simmer for approximately 5 more minutes to brown the lamb and soften the onions. After trimming any extra fat, reduce the heat to medium and add 1 teaspoon of lemon zest, 1/2 teaspoon of dried oregano, 1/2 teaspoon of garlic powder, 1 teaspoon of salt, and 12 teaspoons of black pepper, whisking to combine. Pour a mixture of lemon juice and water measuring 1/4 cup into a shallow dish, then place the lamb in it. Once virtually all of the liquid has been absorbed, continue simmering for another minute or two before whisking in the last 1/4 cup. Add the liquid gradually, about a quarter of a cup at a time, until it is gone. All in all, you should budget 30 minutes for this. The meat should seem damp but not swim in liquid.

- To create the feta sauce while the meat is cooking, combine the yogurt, feta cheese, one tablespoon of lemon juice, one-fourth of a teaspoon of dried oregano, one-fourth of a teaspoon of garlic powder, and one-fourth of a teaspoon of lemon zest in a blender. Combing and processing until uniform. Once the purée is smooth, season it to taste with salt and pepper. Putting aside

- Heat up some pita bread and fill it with the lamb mixture. Drizzle the feta sauce over the dish just before serving.

Recipe : Spaghetti Squash

Prep Time : 0 Hour 30 Minutes

Total Time : 01 Hour 36 Minutes

Yields: 6   Servings

Material :

- Squash for spaghetti, peeled and chopped in half
  Exactly 1 cup of water.
  a half-teaspoon olive oil
- You'll need 1 pound of chicken tenders to make this recipe.
- one medium-sized chopped sweet onion
- 6 garlic cloves, chopped
- Pepper to taste, at least 1 teaspoon
- Artichoke hearts (one can, 15 ounces worth), drained and chopped
- Half a red bell pepper, chopped
- One dried teaspoon of oregano.
- 1/4 of a fresh basil leaf
- One-half milliliter of thyme powder.
- Parmesan cheese, grated (one cup's worth).

Step :

- The oven has to be heated to 350 degrees Fahrenheit (175 degrees C).
  Place the spaghetti squash halves, cut-side down, on a baking dish. Put water around the squash and let it sit.

- It should take around 45 minutes in a preheated oven to cook the veggies so that they are tender when probed with a fork. After 5–10 minutes, it should be cold enough to handle. Use a scraper to get rid of the seeds and then discard them. Pull the meat apart into threads with a fork.
- Preheat 1 tablespoon of olive oil in a large skillet over medium heat. Once the chicken has been added, cook it for about three minutes on each side over medium heat, stirring often.
- One extra tablespoon of olive oil should be heated in a saucepan over medium heat. It is expected that after 5 minutes of heating and stirring, the onion, garlic, and hot sauce will have softened and become more manageable. Squash, artichoke hearts, and red bell peppers should all be mixed together. Flavor it up with some fresh herbs like oregano, basil, and thyme.
- The chicken and Parmesan should be combined in the cooking pot. For approximately five minutes more, while stirring occasionally, cover and simmer over low heat to let the flavors combine.

Recipe : Tuna Bites

Prep Time : 0 Hour 20 Minutes

Total Time : 0 Hour 20 Minutes

Yields: 4 Servings

Material :

- The equivalent of one teaspoon of Dijon mustard
  2 tablespoons lime juice 1 teaspoon grated lime peel
- 1/2 teaspoon sugar
- 2 tablespoons olive oil
- ground kosher salt and black pepper.
- One five-ounce can of white albacore tuna in water, drained and broken up into bits.
- Roma tomatoes, diced, 2 teaspoons
- Red onion, minced, 1.5 tablespoons.
- 1 cucumber, 1 seeded, skinned, and diced, and a pinch of salt.
- The equivalent of one tablespoon of chopped fresh parsley
- Optional: 1 teaspoon
- Eight individual servings of Original Snack Factory® Pretzel Crisps® are included in the package.
- Kalamata olives, sliced and pitted, 8
- Crumbled feta cheese

Step :

- Dijon mustard, sugar, and the juice and zest of one lime are mixed together in a bowl. Blend the ingredients together by stirring. Slowly stream in the olive oil while whisking, and keep going until the dressing has thickened somewhat. Add pepper and salt to taste and combine.
- You may save the tuna in a dish for later. Carefully combine the tomatoes, red onion, cucumbers, parsley, and capers.
-

  The tuna mixture should be topped with the dressing. mildly mixed so as not to shred the tuna.
- Spread some tuna on a pretzel crisp, then layer on some olive slices and feta cheese crumbles for a tasty appetizer.

Recipe : Seafood soup (Mediterranean Seafood Soup)

Prep Time : 0 Hour 15 Minutes

Total Time : 01 Hour5 Minutes

Yields: 5 Servings

Material :

- A pound of prawns and an ounce of cod.
  one onion, cut into quarters
- 1 carrot, peeled and sliced
- 1 celery stalk, finely chopped
- Freshly ground black pepper and salt to taste.
- enough water to drown everything.
- About 6 teaspoons of pure olive oil
- 12 of a small onion, sliced
- You'll need 1 red pepper, diced and stored separately.
- garlic clove, minced
- White wine, dry, half a glass.
- A pound of tomatoes, chopped
- a half-pound of whole clams, prepared and ready to cook
- 12 pounds of cleaned and de-bearded mussels
- At least 4 pieces of bread, more if desired.
- One clove of garlic, halved
- It comes with 1 bunch of fresh parsley that has been chopped.

Step :

- Cod should be portioned up, and the offal should be frozen for later use. You should peel and devein prawns, but save the shells and any other leftovers for another use.
Mix the remaining fish and prawn pieces with the quartered onion, carrot, and celery in a large pot. Add salt and pepper to taste, and cover with water. Bring to a boil, then reduce the heat to low and simmer for 15 to 20 minutes, or until the fish stock has developed a pleasant scent.
- Cut the fish into pieces and set part of it aside. In a pan, heat the olive oil over medium heat. Simmer the sliced onion, red chile pepper, and minced garlic for 5–10 minutes, until the onion and pepper are soft.
-
Add the wine and let it simmer for five minutes. Once the mixture is hot, toss in the tomatoes and bring to a boil. Put in 1 cup of fish stock and seafood like cod, shrimp, prawns, and shellfish. Let it simmer for 15–20 minutes, or until the fish is opaque all the way through and the shellfish have opened.
- Put some bread in the toaster and heat it up. The bread is toasted, and then the garlic halves are rubbed on one side.
- Each serving bowl should have a slice of toasted bread at the bottom. To serve, ladle the soup onto the toasted bread and sprinkle with parsley.

Recipe : Chicken Thighs Mediterranean-Style

Prep Time : 0 Hour 5 Minutes

Total Time : 0 Hour 50 Minutes

Yields: 4 Servings

Material :

- To taste, add sea salt and powdered black pepper to 4 large chicken thighs, bones in and skin on, plus extra thighs to taste
Olive oil, 1 tablespoon's worth
- The Chicken Soup Recipe: 1 Cup
- 6 slices of 1 medium-sized lemon.
- the equivalent of two dried and fresh rosemary sprigs

Step :

- Raise your oven's temperature to 350 degrees Fahrenheit (175 degrees Celsius).
- Make sure the chicken thighs are completely dry with paper towels before seasoning them with salt and pepper.
- In a large oven-safe pan, heat the oil over medium heat. The chicken should be inserted skin-side down into the hot oil. Browning and crisping the skin during a sear should take between 5 and 7 minutes. After a further 5 minutes, turn it over to brown the other side. Remove the skillet from the heat and discard the collected fat.

- Place the pan back on the burner and turn the heat up to medium-high. The meal would benefit from the addition of chicken stock, lemon slices, and rosemary sprigs. Store any extra lemon wedges in the fridge until ready to use. Bring to a boil, then turn off the heat and set aside.
- When ready, reheat the skillet in the oven while covered. The chicken should be fully cooked after around 30

minutes in the oven, at which point the flesh should no longer be pink and the juices should run clear. A thermometer taken from the middle should give an instant reading of at least 165 degrees Fahrenheit (74 degrees C).

- When the chicken is done, take it out of the oven and immediately squeeze the two warm lemon wedges over it. Transfer to a serving plate and garnish with more lemon wedges.

Recipe : Spicy Quinoa Salad

Prep Time : 0 Hour 20 Minutes

Total Time : 0 Hour 45 Minutes

Yields: 4 Servings

Material :

- 2 tablespoons of oil of any kind.
  2 tablespoons of chopped onion.
  pepper, green, one, seeded and diced.
- 1 red bell pepper, seeded and sliced into small pieces
- 1 yellow bell pepper, chopped and seeded
- Chop or crush 2 cloves of garlic.
- 34 cups of quinoa, raw
- Vegetable stock, or broth, enough to fill 4 cups
- One teaspoon of tomato paste.
- Three tomatoes, peeled, seeded, and chopped in advance.
- Italian seasonings tailored to your tastes

Step :

- Warm the oil in a large skillet over moderate heat. The onions and red, green, and yellow peppers should be added after about 5 minutes of heating and stirring. Simmer for a further two minutes after adding the garlic. The quinoa, tomato puree, and vegetable stock should all be combined and stirred together.

- Simmer, covered, over low heat for approximately 20 minutes, or until the quinoa grains are soft, after returning to a boil. Add the chopped tomatoes and some Italian spice and stir it all together. To serve, heat it up until it's piping hot.

Recipe : Med-flounder

Prep Time : 0 Hour 15 Minutes

Total Time : 0 Hour 45 Minutes

Yields: 4 Servings

Material :

- I would want five plum (roma) tomatoes.
  Extra-virgin olive oil, 2 teaspoons
  Twelve chopped Spanish onions
- Two minced garlic cloves.
- Use just a pinch of Italian seasoning.
- In their shells, 24 Kalamata olives, chopped and pitted.
- A splash of dry white wine, about a quarter ounce,
- One-fourth cup of capers
- Freshly squeezed lemon juice, 1 milliliter
- Chopping six sprigs of fresh basil
- Grated Parmesan cheese equals around 1.5 tablespoons.
- flounder fillets weighing 1 pound.
- The 6 fresh basil leaves should be torn and kept aside.

Step :

- Set the oven temperature to 425 degrees F. (220 degrees C).

- Start by bringing a pot of water to a full boil. As soon as the water comes to a boil, take the tomatoes out and put them in a dish of cold water to stop the cooking process. Tossing the skins of tomatoes is a good idea. Prepare the tomatoes by chopping them and setting them aside.
- For about 5 minutes, while the oil is heating, sauté the onion over medium heat until it is tender. Cook for another 5–7 minutes, stirring occasionally, until the tomatoes are tender, after adding the tomatoes, garlic, and Italian seasoning. In a large bowl, mix together the olives, wine, capers, lemon juice, and half of the basil. Harmonize everything together. Turn the heat down to low, whisk in the Parmesan cheese, and simmer for another 15 minutes, or until the sauce has thickened.
- The flounder should be baked in a shallow dish. Cover the fillets with sauce, then top with the remaining basil leaves.
- Fish should be cooked for 12 minutes in a preheated oven, or until it flakes readily when tested with a fork.

Recipe : Pasta from the Mediterranean

Prep Time : 0 Hour 15 Minutes

Total Time : 0 Hour 40 Minutes

Yields: 4 Servings

Material :

- The linguine pasta comes in a single package (weighing in at 8 ounces)
  with a total of three pieces of bacon.
  diced cooked boneless chicken breasts weighing one pound
- seasoned with salt.
- Tomatoes, diced, in their own liquid, canned, 14.5 ounces
- a half milligram ground nutmeg
- One-third of a cup of feta cheese, crumbled.
- 2/3 cup of pitted black olives
- One 6-ounce can of artichoke hearts, drained and

Step :

- Start by bringing a large pot of lightly salted water to a boil. The linguine is done when it is firm to the bite, after 8 to 10 minutes of cooking time.
- Toss the bacon into a large, deep pan. Brown evenly over a medium-high heat source. Once

the meat has drained, you may shred it and set it aside.

- Before you cook the chicken, make sure it has been well salted. Chicken and bacon may be combined in a big pan or saucepan and stirred together. When you add the tomatoes and rosemary, you should keep the pot on high heat for another 20 minutes. The artichoke hearts, olives, and feta cheese should be combined and heated through after being stirred into the pan. Toss in hot, freshly prepared spaghetti and serve immediately. If you want, crumble some more feta cheese on top.

Recipe : Casserole Mediterranean

Prep Time : 0 Hour 15 Minutes

Total Time : 0 Hour 55 Minutes

Yields: 4 Servings

Material :

- 1 kilogram of potatoes
  Extra-virgin olive oil, 3 teaspoons
  Four sardine cans (4.375 ounces each), drained
- Around 500 grams of chopped cherry tomatoes
- Two minced garlic cloves.
- 1.25 grams of dried basil
- Breadcrumbs amounting to 2 tablespoons

Step :

- Bring a large pot of salted water to a boil, then
  add the potatoes. Once it boils, reduce the heat
  to medium-low, cover, and let the veggies
  simmer for approximately 20 minutes, or until
  they are tender. Drain. In order to cool it down,
  cover it with cold water and let it sit for some
  time, being sure to drain and refill the cold
  water as needed. Potatoes should be peeled and
  sliced extremely thinly before cooking.
  To get ready for baking, set the oven
  temperature to 350 degrees Fahrenheit (175
  degrees Celsius).
- The casserole dish should be greased with olive
  oil. Place a single layer of potato slices at the

bottom of the casserole dish. Arrange sardine fillets on top of the potato pieces. Spread a layer of chopped tomatoes over the sardines. Toss everything together and sprinkle with bread crumbs on top of the tomatoes.

It should take around 20 minutes in a preheated oven to cook the dish thoroughly.

Recipe : Mediterranean Roasted Vegetables

Prep Time : 0 Hour 30 Minutes

Total Time : 01 Hour 5 Minutes

Yields: 4 Servings

Material :

- Toss in 12 halved cherry tomatoes Chopped 12 cherry tomatoes Two peppers, one red and one yellow, chopped
- 1 green bell pepper, chopped
- Two zucchini, sliced
- 2-2 medium-sized red onions, quartered
- Prepare two garlic cloves by crushing and peeling them, then setting them aside.
- 2 tablespoons olive oil
- Chopped fresh basil leaves equal one teaspoon.
- freshly ground black pepper.

Step :

- Raise your oven's temperature to 350 degrees Fahrenheit (175 degrees Celsius).
- Put the vegetables in a single layer on a large rimmed baking sheet: cherry tomatoes, bell peppers, zucchini, red onions, and garlic. When serving, olive oil should be poured over the top and stirred in. Black pepper and basil together make for an excellent seasoning.

- Vegetables need to be baked for 35 to 40 minutes in a preheated oven until they are tender and lightly browned.

Recipe : Vegetable Rice Salad

Prep Time : 0 Hour 20 Minutes

Total Time : 0 Hour 45 Minutes

Yields: 4   Servings

Material :

- water, around 4 ounces' worth
  Uncooked white rice measures 2 cups.
  1 & 1/2 teaspoons salt1 1/2 teaspoons cayenne
  pepper2 tablespoons of extra-virgin olive oil.
- 1/4 of a teaspoon of seasoned salt.
- Capers, chopped (one tablespoon's worth),
- 1 freshly chopped fresh parsley sprig
- half a lemon, only the zest
- Three zucchini, peeled and shredded.
- Two carrots, processed until shredded.
- sliced into 12 pieces, a yellow bell pepper
- Cubed and chopped (12) red bell peppers
- The juice of one lemon
- seasoned with salt.

Step :

- Bring the water and rice to a boil in a separate
  saucepan.The rice is done when all the liquid
  has been absorbed and it has simmered for 18
  to 20 minutes on medium heat with a lid on the
  pot. After the rice has finished cooking, remove
  the pan from the heat and cover it with a large

amount of cool water. For a refreshing cold, mix the ingredients together. Put the rice in a bowl when it has been well drained. Use a pinch of herb salt, season to taste, and mix in a tablespoon of olive oil.

- Mix the capers, parsley, and lemon zest in a small bowl before adding them to the rice. Toss in some carrots, zucchini, and red and yellow peppers, as well. One more tablespoon of olive oil, the juice of one lemon, and a pinch of salt will round off the seasoning.

Recipe : Orzo salad recipe

Prep Time : 0 Hour 10 Minutes

Total Time : 0 Hour 55 Minutes

Yields: 4 Servings

Material :

- A half-cup of uncooked orzo
  Ingredients: 1/4 cup of sliced black olives, 1 to
  12 tablespoons of olive oil flavored with lemon,
- A quarter cup of chopped, marinated artichoke
  hearts
- One-fourth cup of canned chickpeas
- A quarter cup of roasted red peppers, drained
  and chopped.
- Pine nuts, toasted, 2 tablespoons
- The equivalent of 2 tablespoons of ricotta salata
  cheese, either crumbled or shaved.

Step :

- Start by bringing a large pot of lightly salted
  water to a boil. When cooking orzo, the water
  should be at a rolling boil, with stirring every so
  often, for about 11 minutes, until the pasta is
  tender but retains a little crunch. good drainage.
- Lemon-infused olive oil is tossed with orzo.
  Throw in some roasted red peppers, some
  olives, some artichoke hearts, some chickpeas,
  some pine nuts, and some ricotta salata. Toss

everything together well. Put it in the fridge so that the flavors may blend as it cools down.

Recipe : Mediterranean Pizza Dip

Prep Time : 0 Hour 10 Minutes

Total Time : 0 Hour 35 Minutes

Yields: 8 Servings

Material :

- Eight ounces of chopped, softened cream cheese from one container.
  8 ounces of shredded Monterey Jack cheese; 1 cup of diced cherry tomatoes; one cup's worth of diced, boneless ham steak; 0.5 cups of drained, sliced black olives.
- 12 cups of marinated, drained, and chopped artichoke hearts 3 ounces of crumbled feta cheese 3 whole, squeezed garlic cloves.
  Fresh basil, chopped (about half a teaspoon's worth)
- A pinch of Italian seasoning, 1 milligram.

Step :

- Monterey Jack, cream cheeseJack cheese, cherry tomatoes, ham steak, olives, artichoke hearts, feta cheese, garlic, basil, and Italian seasoning are mixed together in a bowl. To ensure uniform distribution, stir well. Put the ingredients in an aluminum-covered glass baking dish that can hold 1 3/4 quarts.
- One cup of water should be placed in the insert of a multi-functional pressure cooker (such as

an Instant Pot®). Set the baking dish on top of the metal trivet and place it inside. Replace it and again check the lock. You should use manual pressure and a stopwatch for 10 minutes. Ten to fifteen minutes is about right for the pressure to peak.

- After around 5 minutes, using the quick-release mechanism in line with the manufacturer's instructions, you may slowly relieve the pressure. Turn the key and remove the lid. Stir together and serve immediately.

Recipe : Trout Mediterranean

Prep Time : 0 Hour 20 Minutes

Total Time : 0 Hour 45 Minutes

Yields: 4 Servings

Material :

- You'll need 6 diced potatoes.
  Olive oil, virgin (two teaspoons' worth)
  Four fillets of trout
- Italian seasoning, dry, 2 teaspoons (2 teaspoons water).
- The right amount of salt and freshly ground black pepper.
- 1 very thinly sliced yellow bell pepper (optional).
- 2 onions, medium size, sliced paper thin
- You will need three chopped anchovy fillets.
- A couple of teaspoons of chopped kalamata olives
- The seeds and cores have been removed from four tomatoes before they were diced.
- A single tablespoon of drained capers
- 1 bunch of chopped Italian flat-leaf parsley.
- 2 milliliters of dry white wine.

Step :

- Prepare the potatoes by placing them in a medium-sized saucepan and covering them with water. Once the water comes to a boil, add some salt to taste. Bring to a boil and keep cooking for another 8 minutes, or until the veggies are tender when pierced with a fork. Just dump everything out, cover it, and set it aside.

- While the potatoes are boiling, heat a generous amount of extra-virgin olive oil over medium heat in a large skillet. After that, you need to wash and dry the trout fillets. Add the dry Italian spice combination to the salt and pepper when seasoning the fish. Once the oil is hot, gently add the trout fillets and let them alone in the pan for 10 minutes.

- Carefully switch the fried fillets around. Five minutes after you've piled the bell pepper and onions above the fish, turn the heat back on and finish cooking the fish. At this stage, you may top the fillets with the anchovies, capers, and parsley. Continue cooking the meal at a moderate simmer for another 5 minutes after adding the white wine. Prepare a bed of mashed potatoes and top it with the grilled fish and prepared vegetables.

Recipe : Greek Salad from the Mediterranean

Prep Time : 0 Hour 10 Minutes

Total Time : 0 Hour 10 Minutes

Yields: 8 Servings

Material :

- In a dish, slice 3 cucumbers after removing the seeds.
  Crumbled feta cheese, between 1 and 12 cups.
  black olives, one cup's worth, pitted and chopped;
- Three cups of chopped roma tomatoes,
- 13 cup chopped sun-dried tomatoes; use store-bought ones that came in oil; drain and reserve oil
- Twelve thinly sliced red onions

Step :

- Make a big salad by mixing together cucumbers, feta cheese, olives, roma tomatoes, sun-dried tomatoes, red onion, and 2 tablespoons of the oil from the sun-dried tomatoes. Throw everything into one big bowl to mix. Put in the fridge and serve chilled.

Recipe : Lentil salad

Prep Time : 0 Hour 10 Minutes

Total Time : 0 Hour 30 Minutes

Yields: 8   Servings

Material :

- Brown lentils, dried and measured to one cup.
  Carrots, chopped (1 cup)
  One cup of finely diced red onion.
- 2 garlic cloves, minced or chopped
- There is only enough for one bay leaf in this sentence.
- 1/2 milliliter dried thyme
- Lemon juice, 2 tablespoons
- 1/4 cup of chopped onion
- 14 cup parsley, chopped
- Just a pinch of salt, one teaspoon.
- One-fourth of a teaspoon of ground black pepper.
- About a quarter cup of olive oil,

Step :

- Add the bay leaf and thyme to the saucepan with the lentils, carrots, onion, and garlic. In order to get a depth of 1 inch, add enough water to cover. Reduce heat to low, cover, and cook for 15-20 minutes, stirring occasionally, until lentils are tender but not mushy.

- Once the bay leaf has been removed, the lentils and vegetables may be drained. Adding celery, parsley, salt, pepper, olive oil, and lemon juice will make a delicious side dish. Combine well, and let it stand at room temperature for a while before serving.

Recipe : Mediterranean-roasted vegetables

Prep Time : 0 Hour 15 Minutes

Total Time : 01 Hour 25 Minutes

Yields: 4 Servings

Material :

- Dice 6 large potatoes.
  Red bell peppers, chopped; fennel bulb, chopped; total, 2
- 1.one zucchini, diced
- There are 6 garlic cloves total.
- A generous 6 teaspoons of olive oil.
- 2 teaspoons seasoning
- Vegetable bouillon powder, 2 teaspoons
- Fresh, chopped rosemary, 14 cups
- Half a Cup of Balsamic Vinegar

Step :

- Raise the oven temperature to 400 degrees Fahrenheit (200 degrees Celsius).
- Throw the potatoes, peppers, fennel, zucchini, and garlic into a big baking dish and mix well. Prepared in an oven until the veggies are soft.

Drizzle olive oil over the vegetables so that they are all evenly coated. Season with salt, bouillon powder, and finely chopped fresh rosemary. Give it a good stir and the vegetables will be evenly covered.

- Bake the veggies in a preheated oven, turning them over once or twice, until they are tender. Count on spending about an hour on this. The vegetables should be served immediately after being tossed with balsamic vinegar.

Recipe : Mediterranean-roasted chicken

Prep Time : 0 Hour 25 Minutes

Total Time : 0 Hour 55 Minutes

Yields: 6   Servings

Material :

- sprayed cooking oil
  One 16-ounce jar of four-cheese Alfredo sauce
  Eight tiny red potatoes, halved
- 1 tablespoon fresh lemon juice
- 2 tablespoons butter
- 1/4 tsp. salt.
- About 12 teaspoons of ground black pepper.
- 2.chopped or minced garlic (two cloves)
- 1.25 pounds of boneless, skinless chicken breast halves that have been cut into large chunks
- four Roma plum tomatoes, sliced into quarters
- 4-garlic cloves, crushed and peeled
- 1 tablespoon fresh rosemary, finely chopped
- 12 halved and pitted kalamata olives

Step :

- Raise the oven temperature to 400 degrees Fahrenheit (200 degrees Celsius). Use cooking spray to coat a 9-by-13-inch baking dish.
- Heat the potatoes in the microwave for 2 minutes on high, after placing them in a microwave-safe dish. Then, after 2 minutes on

high, turn the potatoes over while watching for steam. Don't eat the potatoes yet.

- The Alfredo sauce, which should be mixed together in a bowl, consists of lemon juice, olive oil, salt, black pepper, and garlic. Afterwards, arrange the chicken pieces in the prepared baking dish and cover them with the mixture, using approximately a cup of it. Garlic cloves, potatoes, and tomatoes should be arranged in a single layer around the chicken. Dress the veggies with the leftover sauce. The chicken and vegetables should be seasoned with olives and rosemary before being cooked.

- Chicken and potatoes should be baked in a preheated oven for about 25 minutes, or until the chicken is no longer pink in the middle and the potatoes are tender. It's important to cook chicken to an internal temperature of 160 degrees Fahrenheit on an instant-read thermometer (70 degrees C).

Recipe : Mediterranean potatoes

Prep Time : 0 Hour 15 Minutes

Total Time : 01 Hour 0 Minutes

Yields: 16 Servings

Material :

- 2 pounds' worth of potatoes
  Finely chop one green bell pepper.
  1 cucumber (peeled and cut into quarters)
- 1/2 cup red onion, chopped
- Shredded feta cheese equals 8 ounces.
- One lemon's juice
- The Italian salad dressing equivalent of a half cup is
- season with salt and pepper to taste
- Eight slices from three pita breads

Step :

- A big saucepan of salted water should be brought to a boil. For around 15 minutes after adding the potatoes, you should boil them until they are soft but still have their shape. Chop, chill, and drain.
- Potatoes, green peppers, cucumbers, red onions, and cheese should all be mixed together in a big bowl.
- Mix the lemon juice, salad dressing, salt, and pepper together in a bowl. Combine the

187

dressing with the salad and toss to combine. Put out pita bread slices alongside, if you want.

Recipe : Swordfish stuffing

Prep Time : 0 Hour 10 Minutes

Total Time : 0 Hour 35 Minutes

Yields: 3 Servings

Material :

- 8 ounces of swordfish steak (about 2 inches thick)
  2 tablespoons butter
  1 tablespoon fresh lemon juice
- Prepare 2 cups of fresh spinach by washing, drying, and chopping into small pieces.
- Olive oil, 1 teaspoon
- The equivalent of one minced garlic clove is
- one-fourth cup crumbled feta cheese

Step :

- Start with a hot outside grill and a little coating of oil on the grate.
- Using a knife, make a pocket in the steak. Only one side of the pocket should be unzipped.
  Apply a combination of olive oil and lemon juice that has been combined in a cup to both sides of the fish. Leave aside.
  In a small pan, saute the garlic and oil together for one minute over medium heat. Cook the spinach for a couple of minutes in oil to wilt it. Put the food in your pocket and away from the

oven. Fill the pocket with feta and top it with spinach.

- Put the fish on the grill in a single layer and cover it. To ensure the beef is cooked through, turn it over and let it cook for the remaining time.

Recipe : Spice Rub

Prep Time : 0 Hour 5 Minutes

Total Time : 0 Hour 5 Minutes

Yields: 8 Servings

Material :

- 1 pound of sea salt
  Coriander, crushed to a fine powder, 2 tablespoons
  Cinnamon, crushed to a fine powder, 2 tablespoons.
- A ground portion of cumin equals 1 tablespoon.
- 1 tablespoon freshly ground nutmeg
- 1 tablespoon ground black pepper

Step :

- Start by mixing the salt, coriander, cinnamon, cumin, nutmeg, and pepper in a small bowl to produce the spice rub. To preserve freshness, keep it in an airtight container at room temperature, out of direct sunlight.
- Just sprinkle the meat with the spices and put it in the fridge for at least half an hour before grilling or roasting it the way you like.

Recipe : Greek Chicken

Prep Time : 0 Hour 45 Minutes

Total Time : 01 Hour 5 Minutes

Yields: 6 Servings

Material :

- 1 egg
  1/2 cup of whipping cream.
  One cup of crushed saltine crackers.
- 14 cups of freshly grated Parmesan
- 2 teaspoons of finely chopped fresh basil.
- 1 teaspoon of garlic powder.
- season with salt and pepper to taste
- A kilo and a half of chicken thighs without the skin and bones.
- 0.25 ounces of olive oil.

Step :

- Raise the oven temperature to 400 degrees Fahrenheit (200 degrees Celsius).
  In a medium-sized bowl, combine the eggs and heavy cream and whisk vigorously to combine. In a separate medium bowl, mix together the cracker crumbs, cheese, basil, garlic powder, and salt and pepper to taste.
- Remove any dirt or debris from the chicken and pat it dry. Coat each piece in the cracker crumbs mixture, then put it aside after dipping it in the

egg wash. Put the olive oil in a big pan and heat it over medium-high heat until it is just warm to the touch. To get a golden brown color and a crusty texture all over, fry the chicken in the oil for five minutes on each side. Place the chicken in a 9x13-inch baking dish and cover with foil to bake.

- 15 minutes into a 400 F (200 C) oven with the lid on, take it off and let the chicken finish cooking uncovered for another 15 to 20 minutes, or until the juices run clear.

Recipe : Quinoa Salad

Prep Time : 0 Hour 25 Minutes

Total Time : 0 Hour 35 Minutes

Yields: 8 Servings

Material :

- 2 fluid ounces, total of 2 cubes chicken bouillon To make a paste, mash 1 garlic clove.
- 1 tablespoon cooked quinoa
- After cooking, cut 2 large chicken breasts into bite-sized pieces.
- One large red onion, diced and put aside.
- ONE DICED LARGE GREEN BELL PEPPPER
- black olives, pitted and chopped
- Crushed feta cheese is equivalent to 12 cups.
- 14 cups of chopped fresh parsley
- Approximately 14 cups of chopped fresh chives
- a quarter teaspoon of salt
- Juice from two-thirds of a lemon
- 1 tablespoon balsamic vinegar
- 0.25 ounces of olive oil.

Step :

- To make the bouillon, add the water, bouillon cubes, and garlic to a saucepan and bring to a boil. The quinoa is done when it is soft and the water has been absorbed, which should take around 15 to 20 minutes after you add it, toss it in, reduce the heat to medium-low, cover the pot, and simmer it. Put the quinoa in a big bowl, toss in the garlic clove, and serve.

- Combine the quinoa, chicken, onion, bell pepper, olives, feta cheese, parsley, and chives in a medium bowl. Put some salt on it. Marinate the fish in a mixture of lemon juice, balsamic vinegar, and olive oil. Stir the ingredients together well. It may be served either hot or chilled from the fridge.

Recipe : Chicken lemonade

Prep Time : 0 Hour 30 Minutes

Total Time : 01 Hour 30 Minutes

Yields: 4 Servings

Material :

- 0.25 ounces of olive oil.
  2 tsp of freshly squeezed lemon juice.
  2 tb. of grated lemon rind
- I crushed and squeezed four large garlic cloves.
- Dry Oregano, 1 Tablespoon
- one-quarter teaspoon salt
- 12 teaspoons freshly ground black pepper
- It's four boneless, skinless chicken breast halves.
- In this case, we'll need eight little red potatoes, halved lengthwise.
- 1-inch-wide pieces of red bell pepper
- A single red onion, cut into 1-inch-thick wedges,
- a single lemon, thinly sliced

Step :

- Raise the oven temperature to 400 degrees Fahrenheit (200 degrees Celsius).
- Blend together the olive oil, lemon juice, lemon zest, garlic, oregano, salt, and pepper in a bowl. In a baking dish approximately 9 inches by 13 inches, put the chicken breasts. Applying the

lemon juice mixture to the chicken is a must. Collect the potatoes, red pepper, onion, and lemon slices in a bowl. Toss the vegetables with the remaining lemon juice mixture to coat. Arrange the chicken breasts, vegetables, and lemon slices in an oven-safe dish.

- Put everything in a preheated oven and bake for 30 minutes; halfway through baking, spray the chicken and vegetables with the pan juices. Until the chicken is browned all over, the juices flow clear, and an instant-read meat thermometer inserted into the thickest part of the breast reads at least 160 degrees Fahrenheit, continue roasting it for approximately 30 minutes more (70 degrees Celsius).

Recipe : Snow Peas

Prep Time : 0 Hour 10 Minutes

Total Time : 0 Hour 15 Minutes

Yields: 2 Servings

Material :

- To make 1 and a half tablespoons of butter: 1/2 teaspoon of Italian seasoning and 1 chopped garlic clove.
- A 12-pound bag of cleaned and fresh snow peas.
- As much water as you need, starting with 1 tablespoon.
- A single spoonful of pure olive oil
- 1 mL freshly squeezed lemon juice
- Kosher crystal salt with freshly ground black pepper for seasoning.

Step :

- Over medium heat, butter should melt in a pan. To unleash the garlic's scent, add it and boil for about 30 seconds while stirring constantly. Toss the Italian seasoning in with a spoon. Simmer the mixture for another two minutes, stirring occasionally, until the snow peas are bright green and tender. Add some lemon juice and olive oil and whisk to combine. To taste, sprinkle a little salt and pepper on the food just before serving.

Recipe : Tuna Bites

Prep Time : 0 Hour 20 Minutes

Total Time : 0 Hour 20 Minutes

Yields: 4 Servings

Material :

- 2 tablespoons lime juice and 1/2 teaspoon horseradish
  Topping it off with 1 tsp. of lime zest
- 1/2 teaspoon sugar
- 4 teaspoons of butter
- ground kosher salt and black pepper.
- Drain and cut into bite-sized pieces solid white albacore tuna from a five-ounce can packed in water.
- Roma tomato chunks, 2 tbsp.
- 1-1/2 tablespoons of minced red onion
- 1 cucumber, 1 seeded, skinned, and diced, and a pinch of salt.
- One tablespoon of parsley, fresh, chopped;
- capers, a tsp. of which is washed and drained (Optional).
- In this bag of Original Snack Factory® Pretzel Crisps®, you'll find a total of eight of your favorite snacks.
- Kalamata olives, sliced and pitted, 8
- Crumbled feta cheese

Step :

- Mix the Dijon mustard, sugar, and lime juice and zest from one lime in a bowl. Reconstitute by mixing everything together. Slowly stream in the olive oil while continuously whisking until the dressing thickens slightly. Spice it up to your liking by adding some pepper and salt.
- Get a dish and put the tuna in it for later. Add the capers, parsley, red onion, cucumber, and tomato and gently combine.
  The tuna mixture should be topped with the dressing. The tuna should be stirred gently so that it doesn't get chopped up.
- Sprinkle some feta cheese and olive slices over a pretzel crisp and top it with a dab of tuna.

Recipe : Salmon Mediterranean

Prep Time : 0 Hour 10 Minutes

Total Time : 0 Hour 15 Minutes

Yields: 2 Servings

Material :

- Olive oil, 1 teaspoon
  Two fillets of salmon, each weighing around four ounces,
- 4 teaspoons of butter
- The equivalent of one minced garlic clove is
- Twelve cups of chopped tomatoes, or more to taste.
- 1 tablespoon balsamic vinegar
- Here we have six freshly trimmed basil leaves.

Step :

- One teaspoon of olive oil should be heated over medium heat in a small saucepan.
  Approximately 5–7 minutes on each side should be spent cooking the salmon in the hot oil until it is opaque throughout and easily flakes apart when poked with a fork.
- Prepare two teaspoons of olive oil in a separate pan by heating it over medium heat. Stir in the garlic and cook for about a minute, or until the scent develops. Incorporate the tomatoes after around 5 minutes of cooking time and warm

them up. Add the balsamic vinegar to the tomatoes and basil and mix well. Simmer the tomato mixture, stirring it often, for about three minutes, until the flavors have mixed.

- After putting the salmon on a serving tray, put a lot of tomato sauce on top of it.

Recipe : Marinated Mediterranean Chicken

Prep Time : 0 Hour 10 Minutes

Total Time : 0 Hour 15 Minutes

Yields: 4 Servings

Material :

- 1/2 a cup of freshly squeezed lemon juice.
  one-quarter cup virgin olive oil
  Garlic, minced (two cloves' worth)
- 1 tablespoon prepared yellow mustard
- cloves of roasted garlic 1 onion, minced 1
  teaspoon dried red pepper flakes 2 tablespoons
  of ground ore.

Step :

- Combine the oregano, garlic, mustard, and olive
  oil with the lemon juice in a bowl and whisk to
  combine.

Recipe : Tabbouleh

Prep Time : 0 Hour 10 Minutes

Total Time : 0 Hour 15 Minutes

Yields: 5 Servings

Material :

- Uncooked Minute A Multi-Grain Medley is included in this package.
  Vegetable stock, 1 cup
  Approximately 2 teaspoons of olive oil.
- 1 tbsp. of pure, undiluted lemon juice.
- At a ratio of 1 shallot to 1 tablespoon, mince 1 shallot.
- A quarter of a teaspoon of mustard, preferably Dijon,
- Chopped and measured fresh parsley equals 12 cups.
- After peeling, seeding, and chopping half a cucumber, you'll need half a cup of the resulting mixture.
- Cherry tomatoes, halved, half a cup
- 2 green onions, sliced
- 1 tbsp of chopped fresh mint leaves. [Indicative]
- Freshly ground black pepper and salt to taste.
- 1/4 cup of feta cheese, crumbled (optional).

Step :

- Follow the directions on the back of the package for Multi-Grain Medley, using broth for the water called for. Cool.
- In a large bowl, whisk together the olive oil, lemon juice, shallots, and mustard. Combine the other components with the Multi-Grain Medley and stir. A dash of salt and pepper, or to taste, is optional. Feta cheese, if desired, may be sprinkled over top.

Recipe : Pizza Pesto

Prep Time : 0 Hour 10 Minutes

Total Time : 0 Hour 10 Minutes

Yields: 2 Servings

Material :

- 2 teaspoons prepared pesto; 6 inch diameter Greek pita flatbreads; 1/2 cup feta cheese
- The equivalent of 2 small tomatoes, chopped
- About 8 Kalamata olives, pitted

Step :

- Please preheat the oven to 350 degrees Fahrenheit (175 degrees Celsius).
- Spread some pesto over each pita, and then top with sliced feta, tomatoes, and Kalamata olives. Put the pitas on individual baking sheets. Warm an oven to 350 degrees Fahrenheit and bake until the cheese is melted, about 6 to 8 minutes.

Recipe : Lentil salad

Prep Time : 0 Hour 10 Minutes

Total Time : 0 Hour 30 Minutes

Yields: 8 Servings

Material :

- Dry brown lentils to the volume of one cup.
  (1 cup) of carrots, chopped
  There should be one cup of chopped red onion.
- Minced or diced garlic (from 2 cloves)
- One bay leaf
- One-half milliliter of thyme powder.
- Lemon juice, 2 tablespoons
- 1/4 cup of chopped onion
- Minced parsley equaling 1/4 cup
- SALT, 1 TEASPOT.
- a quarter teaspoon ground black pepper
- 1/4 mug of olive oil.

Step :

- Put the bay leaf and thyme in a pot with the lentils and the carrots and the onion and the garlic. Cover it with water to a depth of 1 inch. Bring to a boil, then reduce to a low heat, cover, and simmer for 15-20 minutes, or until lentils are tender but not mushy.
- As a first step, take off the bay leaf and drain the lentils and vegetables. Celery, parsley, salt,

pepper, olive oil, and lemon juice should all be combined. Mix well and set aside at room temperature for a few minutes before serving.

Recipe : Mediterranean-roasted vegetables

Prep Time : 0 Hour 25 Minutes

Total Time : 01 Hour 25 Minutes

Yields: 5 Servings

Material :

- There should be 6 large potatoes, diced.
  2 chopped red bell peppers, 1 chopped fennel bulb
- 1 cup shredded zucchini
- There are 6 garlic cloves total.
- Six Tablespoons of Extra Virgin Olive Oil
- 2.25 grams of salt
- Two Tablespoons of Vegetable Bouillon Powder
- Approximately 14 cups of chopped fresh rosemary.
- Half a Cup of Balsamic Vinegar

Step :

- Prepare for an oven temperature of 400 degrees Fahrenheit (200 degrees C).
- Mix the potatoes, peppers, fennel, zucchini, and garlic together in a large baking dish. Leave it in the oven until the veggies are soft. The

vegetables need an even coating of olive oil. Season with salt, bouillon powder, and fresh rosemary, finely chopped. Stir the mixture to ensure that the vegetables are well submerged.

- For approximately an hour in a hot oven, stirring once or twice. The vegetables should be served immediately after being mixed with balsamic vinegar.

Recipe : Brown Rice Salad

Prep Time : 0 Hour 15 Minutes

Total Time : 01 Hour 0 Minutes

Yields: 6 Servings

Material :

- Between 1 and 12 cups of raw brown rice, 3.0 liters of water one single thinly sliced red bell pepper
- 1 cup thawed green peas
- 1/2 a cup of dried figs
- a quarter of a chopped sweet onion (like Vidalia®)
- Olives, Kalamata, a quarter cup, chopped
- 12 mugs of oil derived from vegetables
- (1/4 cup) of balsamic vinegar.
- 1 and 1/4 teaspoons Dijon mustard
- with freshly ground black pepper and salt to taste.
- 14 cups of crumbled feta

Step :

- The brown rice and water should be brought to a rapid boil in a pot over high heat. Reduce the heat to low, cover, and cook for 45-50 minutes, or until the rice is tender and the liquid has been absorbed.

- Combine the roasted red pepper, frozen peas, dried cranberries, chopped onion, and chopped olives in a bowl.
- Make the balsamic dressing by whisking together vegetable oil, vinegar, and mustard in a separate bowl. shaken vigorously until dissolved.
  Before serving, toss the vegetable mixture with some brown rice and balsamic dressing. To this, salt and freshly ground black pepper should be added.
- Serve brown rice and vegetables topped with crumbled feta.

Recipe : Mediterranean slow-cooker stew

Prep Time : 0 Hour 30 Minutes

Total Time : 08 Hour 30 Minutes

Yields: 10   Servings

Material :

- Diced, seeded, and skinned butternut squash (one).
  The equivalent of 2 cups of eggplant, cut into small cubes and sliced.
  2 cups of zucchini, diced
- Ten ounces of thawed frozen okra
- 1 can (eight ounces) crushed tomatoes
- One ounce of chopped onion, coarsely minced.
- One ripe tomato, cut in
- 1 carrot, thinly sliced
- Vegetable broth, enough to fill a 12-cup measuring cup.
- Approximately a third of a cup of raisins
- 1/2 teaspoon of ground cumin, 1 minced clove of garlic.
- equivalent to 1/2 mg cumin powder
- Turmeric powder, 0.5 milliliters
- one-quarter teaspoon crushed red pepper
- a scant 1/4 teaspoon cinnamon powder
- Paprika, 14 teaspoons.

Step :

- Start with a slow cooker and add the butternut squash, eggplant, zucchini, okra, tomato sauce, onion, tomato, carrot, and broth. Combine the garlic and raisins. Prepared on low heat for 8 hours. including cumin, turmeric, ground red pepper, cinnamon, and paprika.
Cook for 8-10 hours on Low, or until vegetables are fork tender.

Recipe : Tangy tuna salad

Prep Time : 0 Hour 10 Minutes

Total Time : 0 Hour 15 Minutes

Yields: 4   Servings

Material :

- completely pitted and whole Kalamata olives amounting to 1 cup minced garlic, one tablespoon's worth.
  Drain and finely chop 1 teaspoon of capers.
- 3-tablespoons of olive oil
- 5 ounces of tuna packed in water, drained and rinsed.
- 1/3 of a lemon, juiced

Step :

- Olives, garlic, and capers should all be mixed together in the bowl of a food processor. Make a paste by processing the ingredients further. As the blender is running, slowly pour the olive oil in via the feed line and blend until smooth. The tuna and lemon juice are added next, and the mixture is processed until it is totally smooth.

Recipe : Pasta with greens

Prep Time : 0 Hour 15 Minutes

Total Time : 0 Hour 35 Minutes

Yields: 8 Servings

Material :

- 1 (16-ounce) carton of dried fusilli
  Swiss chard, stemmed and in a bunch (1 bunch)
  4 teaspoons of butter
- Sun-dried tomatoes preserved in oil, 12 cups (chopped)
- 0.5 ounces of chopped, pitted Kalamata olives
- Green olives, seeded and chopped, 12 cups.
- One minced garlic clove.
- shredded fresh Parmesan cheese, about a quarter cup.

Step :

- Start by bringing a large pot of lightly salted water to a boil. After incorporating the pasta, cook for ten to twelve minutes, until al dente, and then drain.
- Prepare a microwave-safe dish for the chard. Fill the dish nearly all the way with water. Microwave for 5 minutes on High, or until vegetables are tender, then drain.
- Cooking oil should be heated to a medium temperature in a skillet. Sun-dried tomatoes,

kalamata olives, green olives, and garlic should all be mixed well. You should add some chard to the dish. Put them in a pan with water, and cook, stirring occasionally, until soft. The last step before serving is to toss the spaghetti with the sauce and sprinkle with Parmesan.

Recipe : Onion dip

Prep Time : 0 Hour 15 Minutes

Total Time : 0 Hour 15 Minutes

Yields: 7 Servings

Material :

- Two minced garlic cloves One chopped roasted red pepper one ounce dry onion soup mix
- Twelve cups of crumbled feta
- 1 cream cheese tub (8 ounces each)
- 1/2 cup of sour cream.
- The equivalent of 10 kalamata olives, pitted

Step :

- Utilize a food processor to thoroughly incorporate the garlic, red pepper, onion soup mix, feta cheese, cream cheese, sour cream, and olives. Continue the processing until everything is well blended. The flavors will be best blended if you refrigerate the mixture in a bowl for at least half an hour after you've added them.

Recipe : Mediterranean fish salad

Prep Time : 0 Hour 15 Minutes

Total Time : 0 Hour 30 Minutes

Yields: 6 Servings

Material :

- Dry pasta in the form of little shells, between 1 and 12 cups.
  Three cups of imitation crab or lobster meat.
  Very roughly chopped celery (around 2 sprigs)
- About a quarter cup of black olives
- Mayonnaise, 1.5 c.
- salad dressing, about a third of a cup's worth
- About 2 teaspoons of Worcestershire sauce, or to taste
- Spicy Sauce, One Tablespoon
- 1/4 of a teaspoon of mustard with Dijon seasoning
- Cheddar cheese, one cup sliced.

Step :

- Start by bringing a large pot of lightly salted water to a boil. Pasta should be cooked for another 8–10 minutes after being added to the pot, or until it is al dente. Once the spaghetti has been drained, transfer it to a large serving dish. Using a wooden spoon, combine the crabmeat, celery, and olives. Toss in with mayonnaise,

Catalina dressing, Worcestershire sauce, hot sauce, and Dijon mustard. Add the Cheddar cheese, mix well, and chill for at least one hour, covered.

Recipe : Snow Peas

Prep Time : 0 Hour 15 Minutes

Total Time : 0 Hour 5 Minutes

Yields: 2 Servings

Material :

- About 1.5 tablespoons of butter, a half teaspoon of Italian spice and one chopped garlic clove.
- There are 12 pounds of cleaned and fresh snow peas in the fridge.
- Add 1 tbsp. of water, or more if desired.
- One tablespoon of olive oil, extra-virgin
- Only 1 milliliter of pure, unadulterated lemon juice will do.
- Kosher salt with freshly ground black pepper for seasoning.

Step :

- Over medium heat, butter should melt in a pan. To unleash the garlic's scent, add it and boil for about 30 seconds while stirring constantly. Use a spoon to incorporate the Italian seasoning. Cook the snow peas and water together over low heat, stirring occasionally, for about two minutes, or until the peas are bright green and tender. Then, add some lemon juice and olive oil and mix well. Season with salt and pepper just before serving.